Time's Up

Time's Up

*The Story of My Death, and Learning
What It Means to Live*

Art Townsend

This book is an original production of Beal Road Books, South Dakota.

Copyright @ 2011 by Art Townsend

Cover design by Angela Harwood

Text design by Angela Harwood

All rights reserved

No part of this book may be reproduced, scanned, or distributed in any printed or electronic form without permission.

ISBN: 978-0-615-47383-3

FRONT COVER IMAGES
Blue sky copyright © Rakov Studio, 2011
Pocket watch copyright © Rob Stark, 2011

BACK COVER IMAGE:
Ambulance copyright © Glen Jones, 2011

All cover images used under license from Shutterstock.com.

I would like to dedicate this book to my Father God, without whose grace I would not be here and this book would have never been written.

I also dedicate this book to my loving parents Leo and Anne Townsend. You left this world way too soon but you have always been in my heart. Mom, Dad I'll be home just as soon as this game is over.

CONTENTS

Foreword
viii

Acknowledgments
xiii

Introduction
LIFE IS FRAGILE

3

Chapter One
JUST ANOTHER DAY

8

Chapter Two
HEARTBREAKS

21

Chapter Three
DEPARTURES AND NEW BEGINNINGS

31

Chapter Four
FIRST HEART ATTACK

47

Chapter Five
**PAST BEHAVIOR PREDICTS
FUTURE HEALTH**

61

Chapter Six
YOU CALL THIS RECOVERY?

84

Chapter Seven
IMPLANT + FACEPLANT = TRANSPLANT

105

Chapter Eight
HEALING

119

Chapter Nine
TIME'S UP

133

Chapter Ten
**WHATEVER LIFE I HAVE LEFT,
I WANT TO SPEND IT LIVING**

140

Afterword

163

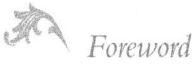 Foreword

These Forewords are from the first responders who saved my life in June of 2009.
—Art Townsend

Many calls that paramedics respond to are cardiac-related, ranging from acute coronary syndromes with myocardial infarctions to cardiac arrhythmias, which can eventually lead to cardiac arrest. With obesity on the rise, heart disease is the leading cause of death in the United States. The American Heart Association estimates that 81.1 million people of all ages in this country are affected by heart disease. There are many causes of heart disease, including congenital heart defects, improper nutrition, smoking, coronary artery disease, diabetes, excessive use of alcohol and caffeine, drug abuse, high blood pressure (hypertension), stress, and valvular heart disease. These statistics show why

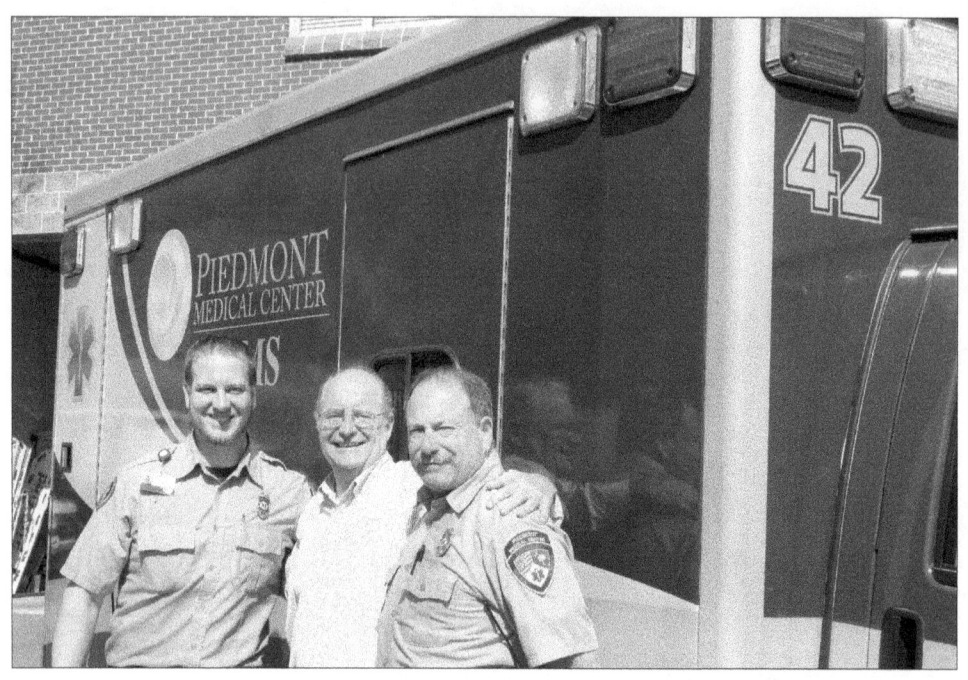

Matthew Hoyle, Art Townsend, and Ricky Benson

the numbers for heart disease are so staggering, and just how important nutritional and lifestyle habits are to overall health.

When paramedics are dispatched to a cardiac call, their minds race with the different cardiac rhythms and their possible treatments. Paramedics use various clues from the scene and, if the patient is able to speak, from the patient to try to find a cause of the cardiac issues. They then piece them together with the medications and interventions used to treat them. The American Heart Association estimates that 95% of all patients who go into cardiac arrest prior to reaching the hospital will not survive; the only hope for these patients is early intervention. It is easy to see that most patients who go into cardiac arrest do not get the opportunity for a second chance at life. On the rare occasion when the interventions performed by the paramedics give the patient a second chance, it gives the paramedics a renewed sense of passion, and it reminds them why they practice emergency medicine.

Matthew A. Hoyle
NREMT-P

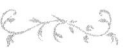

Heart disease not only affects the patient; it also has an effect on the family and loved ones. Lifestyle and behavior changes following a diagnosis need to involve everyone.

Some people are able to live full, normal lives with few limitations on activities, while other people are limited. Things you once did together may be impossible with a life-threatening condition. This doesn't mean you can't do things together. In fact, quality time spent together is part of the prescription, regardless of what you do. Make it count.

For those who have a second chance at life, take full advantage of it.

As a pre-hospital healthcare provider for over thirty years, I have seen too many families wishing for that second chance.

Take the time to look at yourself and your loved ones, and appreciate what you have now.

The clock is ticking.

Ricky Benson
Nationally Registered Paramedic

Acknowledgments

I would like to thank my family who has been impacted by heart disease as much if not more than I have been. You carry the scars the world will never see. Words will never express my thankfulness for your support, encouragement, prayers and most of all your love. Beth, Pat, Randy, Colin, Alice, Isabel, Malachi, Lauren, Matthew, Jorge, Donna, Deborah, Bill and Beth- I love you ALL. The same can be said of my friends and extended family. I would also like to express my sincere gratitude to Pastors Larry Soles and Scott Carroll for your support, friendship and spiritual guidance in my life. I am so honored and blessed to know you. I also would like to say special thanks, at the risk of leaving somebody out, to several folks who went above and beyond the call of duty. Rick, Billy, Chuck & Laurie, Dale & Lisa, Frank, Stephen, Dick, Alan and Page-I owe a debt that will never be repaid! To all the medical Doctors, nurses and staff that performed their duties to near perfection I thank you. To the THOUSANDS of people, most of whom I'll never know or meet, who offered up their prayers for my survival and healing, I humbly say THANK YOU!

In closing I would like to thank Tripper for planting this book seed nearly two years ago. Your encouragement and "kick-start" has resulted in this book. And this would not be a book without the unbelievable organization, planning, wisdom, encouragement and the most wonderful feedback of Betsy Thorpe. I am so thankful for the day Page pointed me in your direction. You have literally been a Godsend and a blessing! I know I have probably left numerous people out but it's only due to my less than perfect memory, but you all know you are in my heart and prayers. God Bless, Art

Time's Up

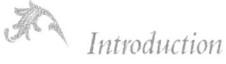
Introduction

LIFE IS FRAGILE

I posted the following entry to my blog on May 5, 2009, nearly one month prior to the date of my death. I never knew how prophetic these words would turn out to be.

Life is Fragile

Those were the words my cardiologist told me on my first visit to his office, following a near fatal heart attack at the age of 37. Life is fragile, and there are no guarantees. As I hear of people dying each day, like Jack Kemp or Angels pitcher Nick Adenhart, I am constantly reminded of that doctor's words nearly 15 years ago.

As we go about our lives and get caught up in "living in the dream," it is very easy to lose focus on just how fragile life is. It usually takes a tragedy or a traumatic event in our lives to wake up and see this reality. For some of us, it might take several events to get our attention. All we have is right now; there are no guarantees on the length of your life. I have a good friend who used to say all the time, "Do you know when you are going to die? Well then, you better start living."

Fortunately, or maybe unfortunately depending on how you look at it, I have had three or four situations where I was either dead or should have died. I died during my first heart attack and was brought back with a couple of jolts from the paddles. I have been in a car wreck, and I got caught in two whirlpools while rafting that could have ended my life. I have also faced personal tragedies with the loss of both of my parents. Despite these life experiences, at times I get caught up in the day-to-day struggles, drama, and frustrations of "life." So I know how easy it is to lose focus of what really is important in this world.

Have your dreams and ambitions, succeed and do your best, develop the habit of going the extra mile, and be who you were meant to be. Remember, all these worldly "things" can be gone in the blink of an eye. Love and relationships are what endure. Both are eternal. Remember, life is fragile. Cherish it, and go live it.

God Bless, Art

I had no clue what life had in store for me a month later. I am so blessed to have another chance to live my life according to God's will, rather than my will. I am so thankful for each day that is given to me. I must admit, though, I still catch myself sometimes fast-forwarding past "now" and thinking, planning, wondering and worrying about tomorrow. I just catch myself much sooner than I did before.

I wrote this book for two reasons. I wanted to tell the story of God's amazing undeserved mercy, grace, and love in my life. I couldn't point to anything in my life that would justify Him giving me another chance. I was not walking in His will. I was not reading His book very often. I had a heart full of unforgiveness. I had not walked the walk or talked the talk. To this day, it completely overwhelms me that I couldn't ask, beg, or plead for His amazing grace when I needed it most. Yet I received it, and this grace, this mercy, this amazing love is available to everyone.

The second reason I wrote this book was my passion and desire to prevent others from repeating the mistakes I made. If just one person changed their attitude, their faith, their eating habits, or their lifestyle, then all the pain and suffering I experienced would be well worth it. If I could get just one person to avoid the mistakes I made, then my life would have some meaning. There is a lot of wisdom in not repeating the mistakes of another.

Life is fragile. There are no guarantees. Most of

us have no idea how much time we will spend on this earth. For some there may be decades left in their hourglasses, and tragically, some may have only a week, a day, or maybe a couple of hours. How much better would this world be if we just remembered how fragile our existence really is? Wouldn't we value things just a little bit differently? Would a house, a car, jewelry, or money have more value than our relationships with our family, friends or strangers? Would we value our eyesight, hearing, touching, smelling or the ability to walk, just a little bit more than all the other "stuff" the world has to offer? What if we really lay our treasures in heaven and focused our sights on the things of heaven, rather than the meaningless things of this world? Wouldn't it be great if we actually appreciated the value of the things in this world that money can't buy? What is the price of love? What is the cost of a relationship? What is our health worth? What is the value of our body? I think the answer to most of these questions would be: priceless. My dad used to always say after an accident or something was broken, "I can always get another car, but I can't get another you."

Einstein said, "Only a life lived for others is a life worthwhile." Do you want to live a worthwhile life? If you do, don't wait until you are on your deathbed to figure it out. My blessing in all of this is the chance to live a worthwhile life. To live that life for others, all you have to do is look at everyone as your brothers and sisters. We are all in this together. Poor, rich, white, black, red, yellow, employed, jobless, homeless, married, divorced, janitor, or president. We are all equal, just different. One is no "better" than another. When I look at others as my brothers and sisters, judgment goes out the window. The key for me is catching myself as soon as judgment enters my mind and remembering we are all brothers and sisters in Christ. Jesus said, *"I tell you the truth, whatever you did for one of the least of these brothers of mine, you did for me." Matthew 25:40*

Writing this book was one of the hardest things I have ever done. Putting words together to express logical thoughts was much more challenging than I had anticipated. Trying to remember events that happened years ago, while therapeutic, was emotional at times. I believe most people want their lives to have meaning, especially as they get closer to the ends of their lives. I am no different. But truly wise people reach that realization at the beginning of the journey. Whether I have two days, two months, or two decades left in this world, I just want to live for today in His will.

In closing, God's grace is available to anybody. You can't earn it or buy it, you can't be good enough or bad enough, rich enough or poor enough. In my case, sometimes you don't even have to ask for it.

Remember, life is fragile. Handle with love.

God Bless, Art

Chapter One

JUST ANOTHER DAY

JUNE 11, 2009

I was born in Mansfield, Ohio, on August 27, 1957, and I died June 11, 2009, in Rock Hill, S.C. I am just an ordinary man with some extraordinary experiences. However, not too many people get the chance to actually write about their death, and for that I am blessed.

For most people, the day they die will be just another day for most folks. The world will keep spinning, people will go to work, kids will go to school and the daily routine will continue unchanged. Your death may be entirely unanticipated, just like mine.

The day started like every other day. I went to work, had a luncheon appointment, and came home for dinner with my daughter, Lauren. After dinner, I asked Lauren if she wanted to go to the YMCA with me. She wisely said. "No," and I'm glad. I know she would have not wanted to witness the upcoming scene. I went off to the Y, unaware that I would not have another coherent moment for a week.

As I can piece it together, here is what happened next. I went to the Y, and around 8:00 p.m. I suffered sudden cardiac arrest (SCA). There is a huge difference between a heart attack and a cardiac arrest - they are not the same! A heart attack is a plumbing issue where an artery in the heart is clogged, which prevents oxygen from getting to the heart muscle. The heart muscle dies or becomes permanently damaged. That is why you hear those in the medical community say, "Time is muscle." A cardiac arrest is an electrical issue where the heart either does not know how, or how fast, to beat. One event (heart attack) is very survivable, and the other (SCA) has about a 5% survival rate (which is reduced 10% for every minute the EMTs are not there).

If you have SCA with no one around, you are dead. Period. The only way to survive SCA is to have someone nearby who can perform CPR or use an AED (Automated External Defibrillator) to shock your heart into a normal rhythm. To actually survive SCA requires a certain series of events to go perfectly, and it requires the right people to be there to help. Missing any one of them will lead to your death. In my mind, the whole process of surviving SCA is a miracle.

The first miracle for me was actually being at the Y where there were a lot of people, rather than at home or by myself. Larry Shields, who I didn't know at the time, but happens to live one block from my house, performed CPR on me. When he tired out, he instructed another gentleman to continue. The EMTs on call that night were Ricky Benson and Matt Hoyle. According to the records, the 911 call was received at 8:20; they were dispatched at 8:23, arrived on the scene at 8:25, and were at my side at 8:27. When they reached me, my initial rhythm was asystole, better known as flat line. They proceeded to start an IV line, intubated me, and in their spare time, shocked me five times between 8:27 and 8:43. Assuming it took the Y approximately five minutes to react and call 911, I was in cardiac arrest for about 32 minutes prior to reaching the hospital. On the ensuing ride to the ER, they regained and lost my pulse three times. I arrived at the ER at around 8:47 p.m. as "Code Blue."

Code Blue is a hospital term used to indicate a patient that needs immediate resuscitation. On TV, this is when the nurses grab the crash cart and start shooting all kinds of medicine into you to start your heart. Then they shout, "Clear!" and whip out the paddles for a large dose of electricity. I like to think of the defibrillation as a taser on steroids. If you like attention in a hospital and don't mind a little electricity running through your body, you will love being Code Blue.

Nobody at the Y knew who I was, because being the thoughtful person I am, I just brought my keys into the Y, along with my iPhone. I had no wallet, no driver's license, and no alert bracelet. Nothing. They managed to figure out who I was, thanks to some smart thinking on someone's part. When you enter the YMCA, there is always a basket for your keys so you don't have to carry them around while you exercise. They distributed everybody's car keys and the only set left was mine, which was brilliant. I had one of those grocery-shopping cards attached to my key ring, and the grocery store just happened to be next to the Y. So they went next door, scanned my card, and found out who I was and where I lived. The modern age of technology came to the rescue again!

As this was happening, an ER nurse pulled my iPhone out of my pocket and saw a text message from my daughter, "Hey Dad, when are you coming home?" This nurse obviously must have been an iPhone user, as she figured out Lauren's phone number and called her. I am positive that this is a phone call no child ever wants to receive. Lauren did what most daughters who love their father would do. She freaked out, had a panic attack, called her mother and aunt, and proceeded to meltdown. Her aunt eventually was able to talk her into driving to the ER.

As family and friends arrived at the ER, Dr. Ramos and a host of nurses worked on me for several more hours. Pastor Larry Soles of the Shield of Faith Church, which was the church my son Matt attended, showed up and immediately began praying life into me, the medical staff, and over all of those who arrived. He returned to the ER numerous times to check on me and my progress, and he continued his much-needed prayers. To survive SCA, it helps to have Pastor Larry praying life into you.

I was shocked 11 more times in the ER (a total of 16 for those keeping count) as they kept losing and regaining my pulse. Finally, at 9:32 p.m., I regained and kept a pulse and normal rhythm. I had had a non-life-sustainable heart rhythm for about 80 minutes, which led to a host of other problems. I was totally unresponsive. I had no eye movement, no gag reflex, no response to pain, nor did I have any eye movement. My only sign of life was triggering the ventilator, which basically means that I was fighting the tube stuck down my throat. I had acute respiratory failure along with pneumonia, and I developed kidney failure over the next several days. My brain was showered with small blood clots from a suspected pulmonary embolism (blood clot) that exploded into smaller pieces during all the defibrillations. These smaller blood clots caused numerous strokes. I was also diagnosed with anoxic encephalopathy, which is brain damage due to a lack of oxygen.

By 11:30 p.m., I was finally stable enough to be transferred to the Intensive Care Unit (ICU). I was put on life support, which means they insert a bunch of tubes in places that shouldn't have tubes, and then they attach the tubes to various contraptions like a breathing machine (ventilator).

My family was told I would remain on life support until Monday, when they would try to wake me up and remove all of the equipment and hoses. The doctors figured my body needed as much rest as possible after all the trauma it had endured. The doctors also told my family, if I did survive, to expect brain damage due to a lack of oxygen and all the strokes I had suffered.

My sister Pat and her husband Randy arrived from Mansfield, Ohio, late Friday and came to the hospital early Saturday morning. That was my third day in the hospital. As they entered the hospital through the double turnstile doors, they met two African-American ladies carrying Bibles. As they reached the elevator doors, my sister held the doors open for them to enter. With their backs to my sister and brother-in-law, one lady repeated all the way up to the third floor, "Jesus is the healer, Jesus is the healer, He will heal." When the elevator doors opened, she continued saying the same thing. As my sister and brother-in-law exited, the other lady looked at my sister and said, "God is a miracle worker, God is a miracle worker. You will see a miracle today." Then they left. My sister looked at her husband, and they were both dumbfounded.

As they walked into the intensive care unit, they looked through the window. They were expecting to see me in a coma. Instead, I was awake and sitting up, with most of the tubes and equipment removed. My sister dropped her purse to the floor and started crying. She could not get the surgical gown on fast enough (all of my visitors were required to wear one). As she entered the room, I said, "What are you doing here?" oblivious to what was going on with me. My sister never saw those ladies again, and to this day she believes in her heart that they were angels.

I have been told that I was very upset on Sunday

night, and Lauren put my iPod on me with the Christian worship group, Jesus Culture, playing. Evidently, I calmed right down. When Lauren re-entered my room a few minutes later, I was singing, "We Exalt Thee," at the top of my lungs. I'm sure everyone in the ICU loved that. There are just some things the good Lord knows you don't need to remember, and my singing would be at the top of the list.

My first memory of the whole event came five or six days later, when my friend, Billy Evans, who is about 6'4" and 275 pounds, visited. He looked me in the eye and asked, "Do you know what an angel looks like?" I stared back at him, wondering why he would ask me such a thing. He repeated his question a couple more times, and I was thinking, "Of course I do. They have these white wings and fly around. And what am I doing here, and where in the world am I?" I realized then I was in a bed that was not my own. This giant I barely recognized had whipped out his iPhone to show me a picture of somebody I didn't know, saying he was an angel. He didn't look like an angel to me. Billy said, "This is an angel, and his name is Larry Shields. He did CPR on you at the Y and saved your life."

I knew right then that Billy had gone back to drinking and drugs. Come on, CPR? I was in the best shape of my life, or so I thought. I was just at the Y working out, so I wondered what I was doing here. It was only a month prior that my cardiologist had told me I had congestive heart failure. I had considered it just another medical term as far as I was concerned, and I just had to work out more often.

It took several days of being told the same thing by my family and friends before I could put all the pieces together. They told me it was like the movie *Groundhog Day* for a week, as my short-term memory was severely taxed. Lauren, bless her heart, made me a calendar for the month of June. She had labeled the various days and what had happened each day. When no one was around, I would just stare at the dates to try to find my memory of that day. But it was all a blank. I have never been more confused in my life than I was with my memory loss. Isn't it funny how God works sometimes? I think there are some things you just don't need to remember. It was such a blessing not to remember being shocked or having tubes in places they shouldn't be.

A few days later, several doctors and nurses came in, wanting to shake my hand and calling me the miracle man. One doctor told me that no one who got shocked 16 times can sit up in bed and actually walk the halls. The neurologist, Dr. Ryder Cook, came in the same day and sat at my bed. He said, "Art, I have been doing this for 30 years and I have never seen this." I asked him what he was talking about. He said they believed I had a large clot in my chest; all the shocks had exploded the clot into a lot of smaller clots, with most of them going to my brain. He said my brain had been showered with those clots, causing numerous strokes. He couldn't explain medically the fact that none of these strokes had caused any long-term damage to my speech, motor skills, etc., except to say it was a miracle. He said most of my clots ended up in the part of the brain that controls short-term memory. I told him that was true. He said I still had two small clots in my brain. One was 9 mm, which had grown from 5 mm just a few days ago. The other one was about 3 cm. He said they would be were monitoring those and expected them to dissolve on their own over time.

I was having a hard time making sense of all this. I had just been at the Y. The respiratory therapist who intubated me came by to meet me, and he said he was glad I was alive. Then he said, with some frustration, that he had intubated me 10 times and that he had never intubated anybody that many times. At that point, I didn't have a clue what intubation was, but I was happy that he had come to visit me.

The next few days passed without anything eventful happening from a medical standpoint. I had a lot of visitors, but unfortunately I hardly remember any of them. Afterwards, one friend told me he had visited me five times during my stay. I told him I couldn't remember any of those visits. He said, "Art, we would have the most lucid conversations for 30 minutes or so. Then on my way home, I would get a text message from you saying, "Dick, did you know I'm in the hospital?" Thank God my short-term memory improved, as I stayed longer in the hospital.

After 10 or 11 days, which in the hospital seems more like a month, all I wanted to do was go home and sleep in my own bed. That's all I could focus on. The cardiologists wanted to put an implantable cardiac defibrillator (ICD) in me to prevent any arrhythmias (irregular heart rhythms) and SCA. I asked them how long it would be in me and they said it would be there for the rest of my life. I didn't want to make that kind of a lifetime decision in the shape I was in. I was exhausted, disoriented, and uncomfortable; I was so tired from sleeping in a strange bed and being awakened every four hours for some routine procedure. All I really wanted was to go home and rest in my own bed, so I could think clearly about putting this device in my chest for the rest of my life.

The doctors wanted to implant this device on Monday and send me home on Tuesday. Sunday night I talked to one the nurses, I think Yurly was her name, who was the largest Mexican woman I've ever met. She was six feet tall and spoke perfect Spanish. We talked for over an hour about the pros and cons of the ICD. After talking to her, I decided to put this procedure on hold and just go home for a few days. I left a voice mail for my cardiologist and said to just discharge me tomorrow, and I'd get back to him on that ICD idea. Yurly came in an hour later and said, "You know, Art, if you go home without that device and have an episode, there is a good chance you will die or become a vegetable before the EMTs get there." I told her she was exactly right, and I had no logical argument against what she said. I called the cardiologist back and left another voice mail to just ignore that last voice mail.

That night I had the best sleep since arriving at the hospital. It was like that deep level 5 REM sleep where you are totally relaxed. But of course, in the middle of night they woke me up to take my blood pressure and temperature. This really upset me because I knew I would not get back to that deep level of sleep. But I rolled over and was able to return to that great sleep level. Later, it could have been two minutes or two hours, I was awakened by Yurly who was squeezing my hand and was right in my face, saying: "Art, stay with me, don't close your eyes, and squeeze my hand." I thought I was still dreaming and was thinking, "Man, I'm really sleeping deeply. This dream is almost real."

I awoke again to a look of terror on Yurly's frightened face and her squeezing my hand, imploring me to look at her and squeeze her hand. I noticed all the lights were on in the room, and my bed was surrounded by what seemed like approximately 30 nurses and doctors. They were all yelling different instructions and shooting medicine into my IV. Not realizing the gravity of the situation (another Code Blue), I looked at the nurses and said, "This is what you have to do to get some attention around here?" I passed out again, only to be awoken by Yurly again. This time I realized it wasn't a dream, and it was actually real. My heart was trying to beat its way out of my chest, and I couldn't breathe very well. The nurses were trying to figure out which ICU had room for me, and they realized I would have to go to the cardiac ICU (CICU) on the first floor. While they readied me for transport downstairs, I realized I had a sudden urge to urinate. As we rushed down the hallways past bathrooms, I asked them to stop so I could relieve myself. Finally one nurse leaned over and said,

"Art, just do it in the bed." I didn't want to do it in the bed, but evidently that's exactly what happened. They were right – in the scheme of things, that wasn't a huge emergency – getting my heart into a good rhythm was.

As the ceiling tiles rushed by and my breathing became more difficult, I think I realized this was a life-and-death situation. I prayed to God, hoping we didn't just survive the last two weeks for me to die like this. Surely there's a bigger plan for me than dying right now. I prayed this prayer over and over. I was also singing the Jesus Culture song, "All I need is you," in my mind. I arrived downstairs in what had to be a Piedmont Medical Center world-record time. They gave me more drugs to stop the arrhythmia. They also put the pads on me to shock my heart again. After a little time passed, I twitched my left leg, and the nurse yelled out "He's out of it!" My heartbeat had dropped from 219 to a normal 70. Then I noticed the pads and realized they planned to shock me again. I was thinking, "No way! I'm awake this time, and I'll feel the shock." I was so relieved to be out of that arrhythmia. At this point, around 5:00 a.m., I was ready for anything they wanted to put in me. I didn't care if it was an ICD, ADD, PMS, CPA, or anything else. I just didn't want to experience another arrhythmia any time soon.

The ICD was implanted that day around 2:00 p.m., and two days later I went home. There were numerous doctors and nurses who did miraculous work to save my life. My family did the work of angels, and for that I will forever be indebted to them. My friends were phenomenal, and I will appreciate their caring and support for the rest of my life.

Nothing can resist the will of God. Even though I was dead, He had other plans. June 11 was just another day. It was the day I died. Fortunately, it was also the day I started living.

 *Chapter Two*

HEARTBREAKS

"Here is a test to find whether your mission on Earth is finished: If you're alive, it isn't."
Richard Bach

Heart disease has been in my life since I was twelve years old. The summer before entering junior high, I played baseball. My father had been our coach for about four years. I always enjoyed baseball, but not as much as my dad did. We ate, drank, and slept baseball throughout most of the year. It was the first game of the season, and I was the starting pitcher. I liked pitching if I had my control, which didn't happen too often. That day, control was nowhere to be found. I hit the first three batters with fastballs, threw an easy groundball over the first basemen's head, and walked the next two. That's when my father proceeded to have his first heart attack.

As Dad lay on the ground, I had no idea what was going on. I figured he had just passed out after the 4th or 5th run crossed the plate. As people crowded around him, somebody went across the street to the fire station. The firemen came over with some oxygen and called an ambulance. My mom joined him in the ambulance for the ride to the hospital, while my sisters and I got a ride with our grandfather. I was really too young to understand what was going on. I was just hoping this might be the end of my pitching career.

In the late 1960s and early 1970s, there was not much technology to treat heart disease. They gave you some morphine for the pain, and maybe some nitroglycerin in hopes that you would pull through. The first 48 hours were the most critical. Children were not allowed on the hospital floors, so we had to stay in the waiting area or hang out in the coffee shop. A child permitted on the floor was usually not a good sign.

My father's prognosis was grim. After a couple of days, we were individually called into his room for our final good-byes. Being the youngest, I was the last one in. I watched both of my sisters' come out with tears in their eyes. My father was my hero, bigger than life to me, but as I walked into his room on this occasion, he seemed much more human. The only thing I remember about our conversation was him saying, "Art, whatever you do in this life, do it the best you can. Otherwise, it is not worth doing." That is great advice when you are doing something good, but unfortunately I also followed it when I did something bad. I left his room with the sense that it wasn't his time to go.

I am the youngest of three children. My parents were Leo and Anne Townsend, and I have two older sisters, Beth and Pat. I grew up in a great neighborhood in Mansfield, Ohio, where all of the neighbors knew each other. There was no knocking on doors, waiting for someone to answer. You just knocked and let yourself in. It was a time of black-and-white TV with three channels, telephone party lines, and no bicycle helmets. Being the youngest of three children and the only boy, I was slightly spoiled (maybe extremely spoiled), very argumentative, and sometimes a little bit cocky. I remember when I was in second grade; my mom told me she hoped I'd be an attorney. I asked her, "Why?" She said, "Because you enjoy arguing so much with others." I immediately replied, "No, I don't!" and started another argument.

I spent most of my time playing whatever sport was in season. In the fall, we played football; in the winter, basketball; and in the spring, baseball. As an athlete, talent and size were never on my side, so I had to rely on discipline and determination. My motivation always started out with a bet. "I bet you can't do _____," and it was on. Our teams were mediocre most of the time, but winning seasons came around every now and then.

I've been a smart aleck my entire life. I got into the usual mischief, and it often started with my mouth. However, as the son of a Marine sergeant, discipline was always prevalent in our house. We were Lutherans and went to church every Sunday come rain, snow, sleet or hail. Being sick didn't get you a pass to stay home. From my perspective, it was pretty much a dead church, as I never saw anyone born again" or witness an alter call, but maybe the adults felt differently.

One particular Sunday, my mouth got me into a lot of trouble. I was 12 or 13, which was almost at the worst of my smart aleck ways. My mother sat on the far inside of the pew. I was sitting next to her, and my two sisters were next to me. My father was on the outside. Mom said something that I can't remember, but my first thought was, "Oh, shut up." Somehow that thought turned to speech, something a wiser person would not have done. I thought that I stopped at "shut" but she obviously heard what I was thinking, and it was on. She proceeded to grab a communion card and start writing. I earnestly wondered what in the world she could be writing. She finished, handed me the card, and sternly said, "Pass this to your father." I turned the card over and read, "Leo, YOUR son just told me to shut up. What are you going to do about it?" I passed the card to my sister, who read it and began to snicker. She passed it on to my other sister, who also read it and snickered. She handed it to my father.

I immediately felt his hand around my neck tighter than a vise grip. To this day, I believe this was the beginning of the Stretch Armstrong doll. Do you remember that wonderful Christmas doll, with extremities that stretched six feet and never snapped? I felt my body rise out of the pew; I prayed this was a spiritual experience and not something manifesting in the physical world.

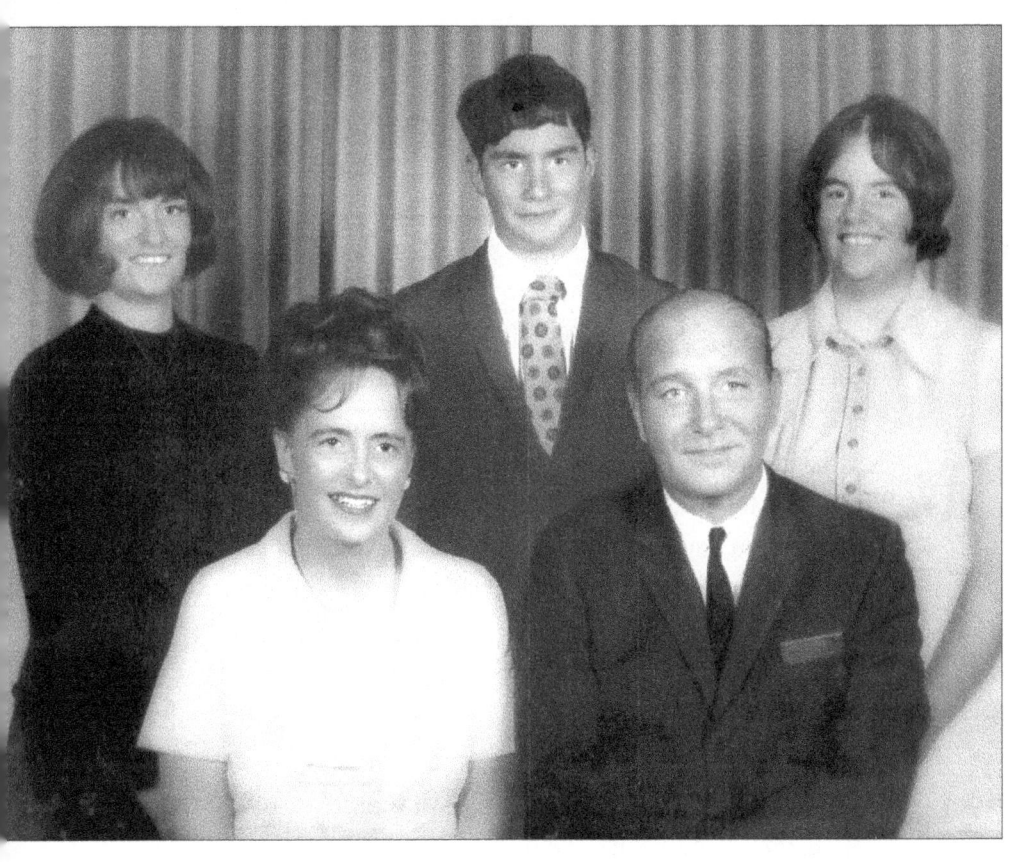

My mom and dad in the front row, and Beth, me and Pat, about 1969. Nice haircut, Art! Where was Photo Shop when you needed it?

Unfortunately for me, it was the latter, and what should have been the Holy Spirit was actually the wrath of one very upset Marine father. As I was hauled down the aisle in front of the whole church before the service actually began, my mind raced with thoughts of what my punishment might be for this slight slip of the tongue.

When we got to the car, I looked at Dad's face and saw it turn shades of red that I never knew existed. I was glad my parents had driven separately, so my sisters would not get to witness this debacle. My father gave me a history lesson on my birth and how the woman I just told to shut up nearly died that day. I tried to correct him, if you can imagine, explaining that it was just "shut" and not actually "shut up." I almost got out of the way of the hand flying in my direction. My dad told me that when we got home, I was to go to the garage and choose a piece of lumber that would be his new, favorite paddle for disciplining his son. Our garage was filled with an assortment of lumber because we were finishing our basement into a rec room. Dad warned that if the board was not large enough, he would pick the next one.

I searched through the 2x4s for something small like a 1x2, even though I knew my dad would reject it. While I was looking, I formulated a foolproof plan. The sooner I started crying, the sooner he would stop hitting me. I made up my mind to just start bawling with the first whack. What a brilliant idea! I spent the next 30 minutes trying to find the perfect piece of wood, praying that it would break in the first couple of hits.

I think you know how this ends. My plan failed

miserably, and my rear end got lit up like a Christmas tree. Needless to say, I never even thought, let alone said, "Shut up," to my mother again.

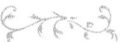

Dad fought back from the heart attack he had the summer I was 12, and he was able to come home. But over the next several years, he suffered more heart attacks and strokes. I grew up looking for the car behind every ambulance to see if I recognized my mother, grandfather or sisters following my dad to the hospital. My mother was a registered nurse and became the breadwinner of the family, as my father ended up on disability. This was a role that placed more stress on my mother than she could tolerate.

We went from being an average, middle-class family to a struggling, one-income family. My sisters eventually joined the work force in high school in order to supplement the family budget. I never noticed that things were tight, so long as there was bologna and ketchup in the refrigerator, and I could play sports. My world was fine. It wasn't until a few years later when Converse "Chuck Taylors" became popular, along with Levis jeans, and I realized that I had neither. My parents had a Sears credit card; if Sears didn't carry it, we didn't get it.

When I was in 8th grade, my family's financial condition became one of the biggest humiliations of my young life. Every Christmas, the student council of our junior high would select a "needy" family in the area and have a food drive for them. One night, the captain of our basketball team, who was also the student body president and one of my closest friends, knocked on our door. From upstairs, I heard my father welcome Steve. The sound of several boxes of food being deposited on the kitchen table alerted me to the purpose of his visit. Steve told my dad that our family had been selected as the "needy" family that year. My dad yelled several times for me to come down and say hi to Steve, but I was so embarrassed and humiliated that I refused. How could we be needy? We lived in a great middle-class neighborhood. My mom and sisters had jobs, and there was always bologna in the refrigerator. Surely there was a more needy family in our town. The rest of my family seemed genuinely grateful for the food, while I hid in my room from shame and embarrassment.

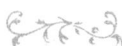

I've always had a problem with authority, whether it came from God, my parents, my sisters, my teachers, etc. There was just something about being told what to do that grated on me. If someone said don't do it, I wanted to do it. If someone told me to do something, I either didn't do it, or I did it unwillingly. Proverbs 16:18 says, "Pride goeth before destruction and a haughty spirit before a fall." That's exactly where mine usually led.

One time, we had a picnic at a roadside park in Ohio with a grill, picnic tables, trees, and gravel parking lot. While my dad grilled the burgers, I decided to start throwing stones at the nearest tree. After a few minutes, my mother told me stop throwing stones before I "put somebody's eye out." I looked straight at her and said, "OK, just one more." The tree I was throwing at was directly in front of me, and my mother was nowhere near it, as I recall. At the time, I didn't know that the stone I would pick up just happened to be the same stone that David used to slay Goliath.

I reached down, grabbed that stone, and threw it as high and as hard as I could at the tree. I wanted to knock that tree down. To this day, I have no earthly explanation as to how that stone ended up right below my mother's eye. I stood there in disbelief as the blood shot out of my mother's face. Upon hearing her screams and cries, my father looked first at his wife, and then back at me. How a person's face can show such deep compassion and anger at the same time is beyond me. Somehow, all the "I'm sorrys" did not take away my mother's pain, nor did it diminish my father's fury. Pride and a haughty spirit will get you every time.

As my dad continued to suffer with heart disease over the years, I mentally prepared myself for his death. I knew it was just a matter of time. I remember staring at his face, just wanting to burn that image in my brain. When he talked, I wondered if I would forget the sound of his voice. With every ambulance siren, I wondered if his life was over. These were not the usual thoughts of a young teenager, but it was my reality.

The sound of my mom screaming in pain awakened me around 6:00 a.m. on March 11, 1974. Dad yelled upstairs that he was taking Mom to the hospital. I went about my normal morning routine, getting ready for school and not worried at all. Other than an ulcer or two, she seemed as healthy as a horse.

I drove to school that day in my own little world of sports and peer pressure. Around 11:00 a.m., I was called down to the principal's office. I immediately wondered if any pranks I had been involved in warranted such attention. Nothing came to mind, so I was clueless when I entered his office. He said that the hospital had called, and I needed to go sign some papers for my mom's surgery. That just didn't make sense to me because I figured my dad was there to take care of things. However, I realized this was a ticket out of school and didn't say a word.

The only surgery I could imagine Mom requiring would have been for her stomach. I grabbed my keys and rushed out to the parking lot. For just a split-second, I had this far-fetched thought that maybe she was dead, but I dismissed it as quickly as it had entered my mind. I turned my attention to how long the hospital visit would take, and what my plans would be for that afternoon. I loved my freedom, and there wasn't much better than being 16 and driving.

I arrived at the hospital and walked into the emergency waiting room. My grandfather, father, and sister were there. Dad talked about what happened between 6:00 a.m. and 10:00 a.m. Our family doctor met them in the emergency room, examined her and sent them home. A little while later, my Mom's pain intensified and they returned to the emergency room. My grandfather, my mom's father, told stories, and I waited patiently to be dismissed.

After what seemed like two hours, our family doctor came in. He was followed by a nurse with a syringe. What he said next changed my world forever. He looked at my father and said, "Leo, I did everything I could to save her." My father shot up out his chair, screaming and crying. The nurse, knowing my dad's cardiac history, immediately gave him a shot in his arm to sedate him. Everyone in the room burst into tears, myself included. I could not believe what I had just heard. Surely this wasn't happening; there was a mistake somewhere. I was in shock, and my world just stopped. There was no way this could be happening. I had never felt so much pain and hurt. My heart felt like it was beating out of my chest. This just couldn't be. For years I had prepared myself for my dad's death, knowing that my mom would always be there. How could this happen? I was dazed, and I stayed that way for a while. What do you do when the world crashes down around you?

I don't remember driving home from the hospital, but I do remember slamming some kitchen cabinet doors in anger once I got home and my sister yelling at me to stop.

I realized that I had not said goodbye to my mom that morning. I hadn't told her I loved her because I knew I'd see her after school. To this day, we don't know what she died of. Our family doctor speculated it was an aortic aneurism, but without an autopsy we wouldn't ever know for sure. I was in my own world, and I took for granted those nearest to me. It was my first lesson that there are no guarantees in life. However, it took quite a few reminders before that lesson actually sank in.

Chapter Three

Departures and New Beginnings

The unexpected death of a loved one, parent, spouse or child, is a shock. The finality is overwhelming. It's not like making a decision, and then realizing it was a bad idea and changing it. There is no "oops" I made a mistake, let me correct it. The idea that you will never see your loved one again in this life is heart shattering. The opportunity to say the things that have been left unsaid for many years is lost forever in this world.

The death of my mother was the defining moment of my life. It changed my life forever. It's almost like my entire life is categorized by what happened before and what happened after her death. Prior to her death, my life seemed perfect, despite the health problems of my father. As long as there was bologna and ketchup in the refrigerator and some sports event to play outside, my world was fine. I felt loved, secure, peace, joy and most of the time – happy.

I was in a haze the whole week of my mom's funeral. Time passed so slowly; all I wanted was the world to stop for just a day and recognize or acknowledge the fact that my mom had died. I just wanted to yell at the top of my lungs, "Hey, stop! My mom just died!" But school stayed open, people went to work and the earth kept spinning. I wanted somebody to tell me why this happened, but it was a question that had no answer. I remember all my relatives showed up, some I hadn't seen in a long time. I know they were there to comfort my father and our family, but I couldn't help wondering why it took a death to bring us all together? Why do we wait for a tragedy to happen to justify a visit?

I was lost. Nothing was ever "normal" again in my life. At 16, I had a hard time comprehending death. I remember for a long time I expected to see Mom every time I turned a corner in our house, and hear her voice reminding me about some chore I needed to do. As time went by, the finality of Mom's death became more and more real. Christmas that year was the lowest point of my life. All the joy and happiness of the holiday was gone forever. I cried a lot those few weeks, most of the time by myself. I was the "man" of the family now and back then men didn't cry, at least that's what I thought. Most of the time I tried to hide my tears and just find some place to be alone. I had never experienced pain so intense before.

I guess this is why I'm so adamant that *Life is Fragile*. Death is an event that usually changes your life forever, and in my case left me with regrets. My only comfort was knowing Mom was in Heaven, and one day I would be able to express to her all the regrets I carried.

The time we have together should be cherished; it shouldn't be taken for granted. Theses are sacred, divine moments; all of them. And most of the time we never realize it until it's too late. We will regret all the words said in anger, and hold on to those spoken out of love, from our heart. And we will wish we had more of the latter.

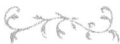

In the year after my mom died, my dad suffered a couple of strokes and endured more hospital stays. We came to the conclusion that he would have to go to a nursing home. My oldest sister, Beth, was in college and my middle sister, Pat, worked during the day. I was in high school, and Dad needed around-the-clock care.

Dad loathed nursing homes and swore he would never live in one. I still remember the afternoon we moved him. The strokes had left him pretty feeble-minded, but as soon as he figured out where we were headed, he tried to bolt from the car. It took everything my next-door neighbor Mike and I had to keep him inside. The next morning, someone from the nursing home called and said he had died. I like to think Dad died of a broken heart, having lost the love of his life when my mom died. I was seventeen and a senior in high school the day he died, which was April 29, 1975.

The death of my father was almost a relief. He had suffered for so many years with heart disease and was in so much pain; I knew he was now in Heaven and free from pain. I remember sitting on the front stoop and one of my uncles said, "You know, Art, you have now faced one of life's greatest tragedies – the loss of your parents." I didn't find much solace in his words at that age, but I knew he was just trying to help. In spite of all of my mental preparation, losing my dad still hurt tremendously.

Over the next several years, I became very angry with God. I must have asked him, "Why?" a thousand times a day. I never got an answer, so I tried making one up. At first, I thought it must have been my fault, and I was being punished for my bad behavior. Then I thought maybe the lesson was to make sure others didn't take their parents for granted. Later, I figured they were needed in Heaven more than they were needed on Earth, as if there are any needs in Heaven. It went on and on.

For the next 34 years, *I* told God what His will was for my life. I told him what I wanted to do, who I wanted to hang out with, and where I wanted to go. I told him how and where I would spend my time, money, and thoughts. I advised God, I argued with God, I instructed God, I corrected God, and I blamed God for all the bad things in my life, while taking credit for all the good things. I convinced myself after my parents' deaths that it was me against the world. Nobody had my back, and there was no safety net. It was up to me to make it or break it.

A good friend of mine has a saying, "Hurt people hurt people, and healed people heal people." I hurt a lot of people over the years. To deal with the pain, I turned to alcohol and running. My dad made me promise him before he died that I would go to college for at least one year. While in college, I started running 3-5 miles a day several times a week, running an eight-minute mile. The pounding of my feet on the pavement helped manage my anger, and the alcohol numbed the pain for a while. I remember my mantra while running was, "I'll never let myself get in the shape of my old man," followed by, "I'll never leave my kids like my parents did."

I graduated from Wittenberg University with a degree in accounting. I think I chose accounting because I liked math, and I knew once I got my CPA certificate, the rest of my life would be blue skies. Did that ever prove to be false! College does a great job of teaching you how to make a living, but it does a horrible job of teaching you how to live.

Finding a job in 1979 was a struggle. I lived in a house with eight other guys, and our walls were posted with rejection letters from every Fortune 500 Company in the Northeast. I was hoping to land a job with one of the "Big Eight" firms. The Big Eight stood for the eight largest public accounting firms in the world. In the accounting world, landing a job with one of them guaranteed blue skies, or so I thought. Today I think it

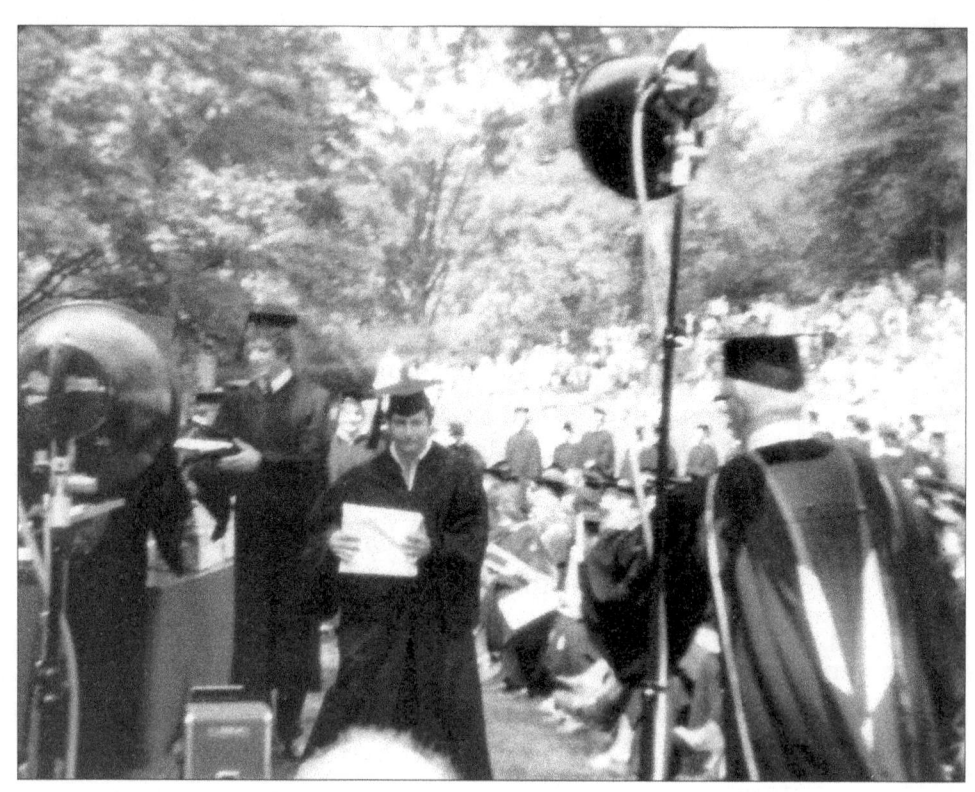

College Graduation, 1979

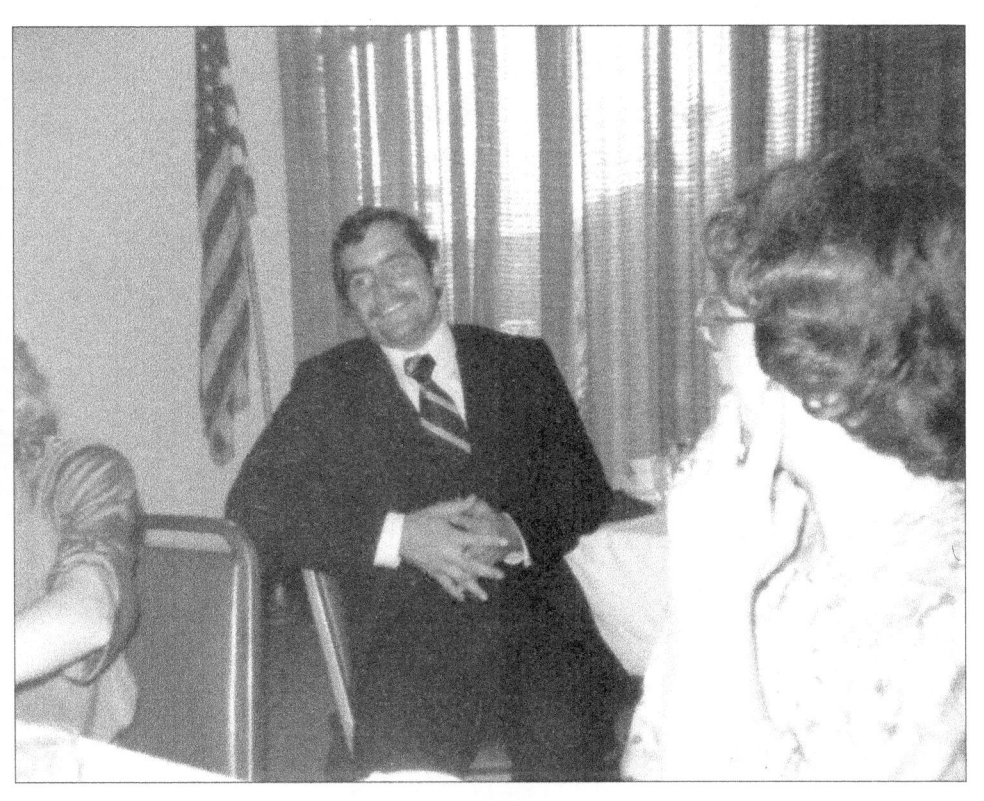

College Graduation Party – About to Join the Real World

has shrunk to the Big Three, thanks to mergers and a shrinking economy. I was rejected by every accounting firm in Ohio, so I turned my job search to the South.

I headed to Charlotte, North Carolina, to visit my sister Beth and her husband for Christmas. In the fall, I decided to send out my resume to all the Big Eight firms in Charlotte. I immediately got seven rejection letters in the mail. The only firm that did not send one was Touché Ross. When I got to Charlotte, I decided to call them and make sure my rejection letter was not in the mail. I called the partner to whom I sent my resume, expecting to be passed off to a secretary. Much to my surprise, the partner, Woody Nail, answered. I told him I had sent him my resume. He replied, "Art, I have a hundred resumes on my desk right now, but if you can come down here at 4:30 p.m., I'll interview you."

I arrived at 4:25 p.m. and mentally went through all of my rehearsed responses and questions. The interview seemed to go well, as I was introduced to several partners and managers. The pecking order in the public accounting world at that time went from junior accountant (grunt) to senior accountant to manager to partner and managing partner (head honcho). I ended up in the conference room at 6:00 p.m. with the managing manager (yes, this is a title, believe it or not), Robert Underwood. Robert asked me what I was doing "down here." When I explained I was visiting my sister and had gotten a job stocking toys at the local Brendle's catalog showroom the day before, he hired me on the spot. He said, "Art, to come down here and get a job in a couple of days impresses me. You must be a go-getter. I am going to recommend that we hire you."

After what seem like an eternity alone in that massive conference room, Woody called me into his office. I sat down and he said, "Boy, Art, you must have impressed a lot of people. We are only hiring two people this year, and I'm happy to tell you that you're one of the two." With that, my life in public accounting began. Everything after that was pretty much a blur, but being an accountant, I do remember the offer was $1,200 a month with a $1,600 guaranteed bonus. Being the math whiz I was, I could total that up without a calculator to an annual salary of $16,000. That was all the money in the world to me back then!

My employment started in August of 1979, and I had nearly eight months to figure out how to spend $1,200 a month. I immediately went back to Ohio and bought a brand new 1979 Mazda RX-7. Of course it was financed, but the payments were only $275 each month, which left me over $925 a month to spend, plus there was a year-end bonus. I picked out a one-bedroom apartment in the most expensive neighborhood in Charlotte at the time, South Park, for only $290 per month. This still left me with $635 a month. So being young, dumb, and without furniture, I of course went to the furniture rental store to pick up a dining room and living room outfit. This cost $175 a month to rent, leaving me still $460 a month. That was plenty of money to buy food, pay insurance and put gas in the car, or so I thought.

Touché Ross had a bi-monthly payroll, which meant I would be paid $600 on the 15th and 30th each month. I couldn't wait for the office manager to hand out paychecks the very first 15th that I worked. She called me into her office and gave me my check. I tore open that envelope, expecting a check for $600.00. The look on my face had to have been priceless when I saw the total of only $412.56. I asked, "Ruth, where is the rest of my money?" She looked at my pay stub, and with love in her eyes, she said, "Art, dear, we have to deduct payroll taxes." All the way back to my cubicle I kept thinking, "Taxes, taxes, taxes. How could I forget about payroll taxes?" I was an accountant! This career was not starting out too well. I sat down in my cube, pulled out my calculator, and quickly realized the $85.12 left after tax was not going to cover car insurance, gas, food, and going out.

I spent four years in the public accounting industry. I worked in what was called the audit division, as opposed to the tax division or consulting division. A client's accounting clerk described it best to me one day when she said, "Art, you are the guys who come in after the battle has been fought, and you stab all the wounded!" That's exactly what we did. Clients always loved the tax division guys because they saved them money, and they despised the audit division guys because we were a big headache.

I learned a lot at Touché Ross. I learned what being "professional" meant, and I gained a work ethic. I met a bunch of really intelligent people who, quite frankly, were never on the short yellow bus where I had spent most of my life. I traveled a lot and, I was exposed to many different industries. I also learned office politics, how to make partner, or rather how not to make partner, and I learned that I didn't want to spend my career in public accounting.

I got married to my future ex-wife in June of 1982. She had a wonderful son from a previous marriage, Colin, and I adopted him shortly after our marriage. We had two more great kids shortly thereafter, Lauren and Matthew. Unfortunately, it took me 18 years to realize that this was not a healthy relationship for anyone involved.

I left public accounting in March of 1983 and accepted the position of controller for Dexter R. Yager, Sr., and his related businesses. At the time, it was a small, family-run private business with less than 100 employees. Having spent four years in the most professional environment imaginable, going to a family-run business was quite a shock to me. Dexter was the largest Amway distributor in the world, and he was one of those people that you either loved or hated; there was no middle ground. I fell on the love side. I worked there five years, but I put in 15 years of work time. I worked all day, late nights, weekends, and holidays. Even when I wasn't there, I was thinking about work. Dexter was one of those guys who gave you all the responsibility you asked for, and I always asked for more.

Being all of 25 and working for one of the most

successful individuals in North Carolina, I knew that all my hard work would pay off financially at some point. I just knew that one day Dexter would walk in and hand me a $10,000 or $20,000 bonus check. What I didn't factor in was Dexter's belief that highly paid Fortune 500 executives were paid about $30,000 a year. In five years, I think I got two raises. But what Dexter poured into my life was worth much more, namely wisdom, faith, and positive thinking. I didn't realize it at the time, but I would carry the things he taught me for the rest of my life.

Most people have heard of Amway or have an Amway story, either good or bad. It was one of the first multi-level marketing companies. Today, I think it is referred to as network marketing. When I worked for Dexter, it was estimated his network of distributors was in the 200,000-300,000 range, and his group generated 1/3 of Amway's total sales. It is even larger today. I have seen figures estimating it to be two to three million distributors. Dexter was the most positive person I have ever met. Publicly or privately, good times or bad, nothing affected Dexter's attitude. I never saw him down, no matter what news I brought him. Trust me, in the mid-1980s there were a lot of negative items to bring him.

Dexter was also the most conservative Christian businessman I have ever met. He was the tea party before there was a tea party. His message has always been God, country, and family in that order. Dexter was a huge man of faith. I remember my first business meeting with him. He called me into a real estate meeting one night with his other two partners. They had purchased a significant tract of land of 400–500 acres in South Charlotte. As I walked into the meeting, they had land surveys rolled out on the conference room table. Their hands were on them, and they were praying out loud. The first thought that raced through my head was, "If the boys at Touché Ross could only see me now." They prayed over the property, asking God to bless this tract of land and make it prosperous. I was highly skeptical, due to my ignorance, and I wondered what I had gotten myself into. They eventually sold the land to one of the largest developers in Charlotte, who in turn developed it into one of the most expensive areas of town called Ballantyne.

Dexter could relate anything to success; this was his main focus for the five years I was around him. One time he wanted me to present a condominium development opportunity to his top distributors. They were out on Lake Wylie on Dexter's houseboat, and he asked me to join them. Most people would have docked the houseboat for me to get on, but not Dexter. He had his oldest son Doyle drive me out in his speedboat to track them down. We spotted Dexter and his houseboat and, instead of stopping, Dexter just motioned us to pull alongside of him. I was in a suit, carrying a briefcase, jumping from one boat to another at about 20 mph. As I entered the living room filled with his top ten distributors and their wives, Dexter was finishing up his talk about how sex was a lot like success. He finished, looked at me, and said, "OK, Art, tell them about that condo deal." I looked at him quizzically and said, "You want me to talk about a real estate deal after that?" Needless to say, not many people were interested in any investments that day.

Outside of people, Dexter only invested in real estate. He did not like the stock market or bonds. He always said, "I don't want to look in the paper every morning to see how much I'm worth. I like sticks and bricks. I can hit the road for a month or two, and when I get back, I know that real estate is still there." It was his love of real estate that landed me my next job in March of 1988.

I accepted the position of CFO for Lat Purser & Associates, Inc. (LPA) in 1988. While it was also privately owned, it enjoyed a very professional reputation with a lot of young, aggressive talent. LPA specialized in the development, leasing, brokerage, financing, and management of grocery-anchored shopping centers. Unfortunately, the first year was marked with a nasty divorce between the two largest shareholders. It took nearly a year to unwind the property ownership, and it was a legal nightmare. The son of the founder, whose name was on the door, remained. I stayed there for 11 years until I was fired in 1999. The owner, Lat Purser, and I could not agree on a commission policy change, and it was my time to leave.

I had received a paycheck for twenty years and had built my lifestyle around that stream of income. I went on several job interviews without much success, and I ended up working for myself. I generated very few fees that first year. The next year, I partnered with a friend of mine who had been a commercial mortgage banker, and we set out to finance commercial real estate.

We proceeded to go broke for the next two years. We didn't generate a dime, and every day I woke up scared, wondering what we were going to do to generate revenue. During this time I also went through a divorce. The kids and I were living in an apartment with inflatable living room furniture and a card table in the dining room. How did I survive? Well, I liquidated my share of my 401k plan, set up a line of credit with the best banker I have ever met, and borrowed from friends when I needed to.

Finally, my 401k ran out, I had tapped out my line of credit, and friends weren't really enthusiastic about loaning me more money. God sent me an epiphany. One day I looked at my partner and said, "You know, Dexter used to always say the crumbs off a rich man's table are better than any meal from a poor man's table. You need to hang out with our richest client 2-3 days a week and just catch the crumbs." At that time, I was past broke. I owed the bank more money than I could ever imagine paying back. That strategy eventually paid off, and we started to close deals, which generated income. It took a few years, but I ended up paying back the bank, my friends, and digging out of that hole.

The two or three years that I was broke taught me

one of the biggest spiritual lessons of my life. <u>Do not worry.</u> Live for today, as that is all we have. Tomorrow has enough worries of its own. As long as there is a roof over my head, food in the refrigerator, and nobody with a gun is demanding money, it is OK right now. As soon as I start to live in the future, worry overwhelms me. When I start having thoughts about what bills are due next month, what will happen if this deal doesn't close, what if so-and-so says this or that, then I know I'm not living for today. Trust me this is easier said than done, especially for a guy who had spent his last 20 years budgeting every dime that came in. I struggle with this even now. I have to consciously remember back to this period in my life and know that God provided for me then and He will get me through this struggle as well. We spend so much of our lives thinking, planning, worrying and focusing about future events, and all we have is right now. And the irony is most of what we worry about never happens.

There is wisdom here. It seems to me the biggest lessons I learn in life usually come with the biggest struggles. I hope you don't have to go broke for two or three years, incurring a lot of debt, to learn to live for today. DO NOT WORRY!

Chapter Four

First Heart Attack

My wife hounded me for the first several years of our marriage to go to the doctor and get a physical. She was always worried, given my family history, that I was a candidate for heart disease. I had probably gained 30-40 lbs. since my college days, exercised very little, ate whatever I liked, and filled my life with the stress of day-to-day living. When I was in my early 30s, I finally gave in and went to see our family doctor. He did a routine physical and took some blood. A week later, he called me back in to go over the results. My blood work showed my cholesterol at 375, which was nearly two hundred points above the suggested 200, my LDL was so high that it could not be measured, my HDL was about 35, and my triglycerides were 2,800 (normal is under 200). I think at this point, my blood was more white (fat) than red. The doctor told me, based on my family history and current lab numbers, it was not "if" I would have a heart attack, but "when." In a few short years, I had become just like my father, and all those years of running had gone to waste.

At this point in his life, a smart man would have made some significant changes. I did make a few, like walking 30 minutes a day and watching what I ate. The doctor assigned me to a dietician. Every two weeks, I had to report for duty with my notepad listing everything I ate, day by day. She examined that notepad with a microscope, interrogating me on my food choices. It didn't take long to get with the program, and I lost 20-30 lbs. over the next several months.

I stayed with the regimen for about a year and then life happened, as it always does. Little by little, I stopped doing things; I stopped seeing the dietician, I stopped walking, and I stopped watching what I ate. Before I knew it, I had not only gained back what I had lost, but I had added another 10 lbs.

Four years since that warning from my physical, I believed I had missed the heart disease bullet. It was September of 1994, and I was 37. It was just another day. In the afternoon, however, I noticed some discomfort in my chest when I walked upstairs. I blamed this sensation on the Chinese food I had eaten for lunch.

The next part is where pride really messed me up. As I left the office and headed to my car, the chest pain increased. I was still in denial and thought the pain was just a bad case of acid indigestion. As I was driving home, I passed three exits, each of which would have

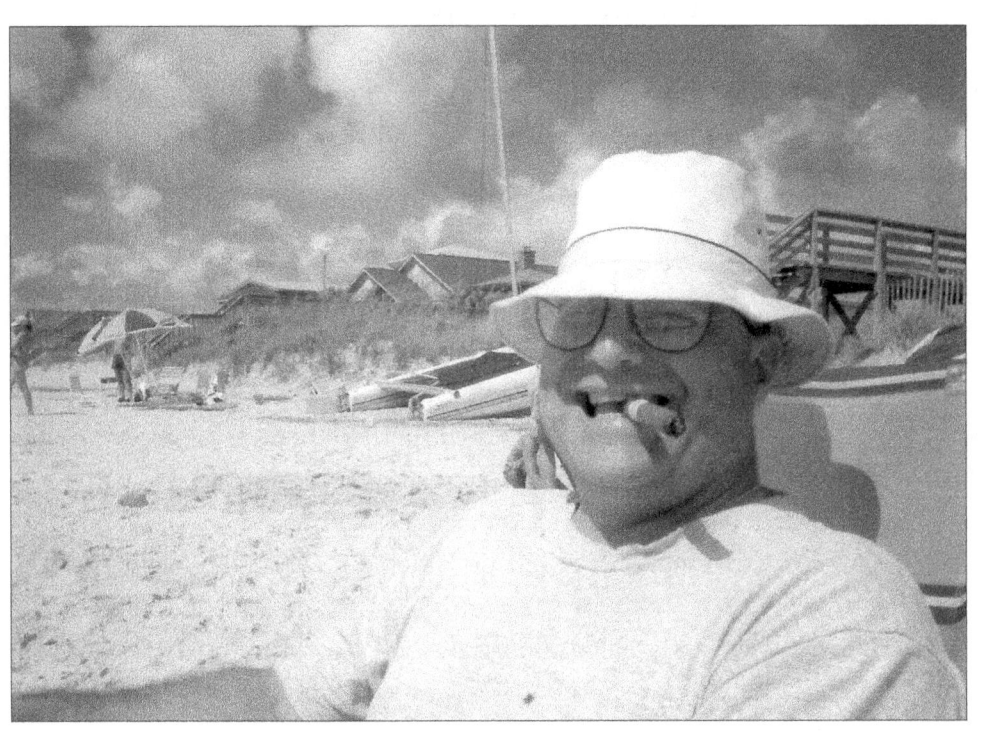

Living Large in the 1980's

led me to a hospital for treatment. I felt like if I could get home and take off my shirt and loosen my belt, I would get some relief. But home was a good 45 minutes away from work, and it was also 30 minutes away from the nearest hospital.

Being the hard-headed, prideful guy I was, I chose to ignore all three of those exits and head home. It was a decision that would have very serious, long-term consequences. As I neared home, the pain became quite intense and also began radiating down my left arm. It was then that I resigned myself to the fact I was having a heart attack, and this was definitely not indigestion.

I decided to call my wife on my new Motorola flip phone. Just as I told her to call an ambulance because I thought I was having a heart attack, I crested a hill, headed down the other side, and the signal was lost. That small incident didn't do much for my stress level.

We lived out in the country at the time, and our driveway was a half-mile of gravel. As I pulled my car into the driveway, my wife was flying out in her car, coming to look for me. At the last instant, we dove in opposite directions, barely avoiding a head-on crash. I continued up to the house, still clinging to the misconception that if I could just take my shirt off, my chest would feel much better. I entered our bedroom, removed my shirt, and lay down on the bed. I was confident that the pain in my chest would subside, and that calling an ambulance was unnecessary. Well, that didn't happen. As I lay down, not only did the pain not subside, it actually increased. It increased so much that it felt like an elephant was sitting on my chest. I had never felt so much pain and pressure in my life.

Fortunately, the EMTs showed up because my wife had called 911. Was I relieved to see them! They wheeled in their stretcher, put the oxygen mask on me, and started an IV. As they rolled me out of the house, I realized I still had my keys and wallet, so I handed them to my wife. Nobody had my ATM pin-code, so the last words after, "I love you," were, "And my pin number is xxxx." Only an accountant would think in those terms!

Once inside the ambulance with the IV in place, the EMT hooked me to an EKG machine. About halfway to the hospital, he gave me a nitroglycerin tablet to put under my tongue. I looked at him and asked, "Do you think I'm having a heart attack?" He said, "No, I don't think so." He probably thought the truth would make things even worse. I told him I was getting light-headed and felt faint, and he told the ambulance driver to go faster. BOOM! Out went the lights, and I passed out. I was immediately out of pain and traveling rapidly through a dark tunnel. I could sense there were people on the side of the tunnel that I was quickly passing through, but I had no time to chat. I also had no idea that I had died, because it seemed I still had all of my senses, as well as the ability to think and reason. Then BOOM again. They had shocked me three times, and in the words of the EMT, "Art, the third time we shocked you, you sat up and said, 'I'm back!'" I don't know about that, but I do remember feeling like somebody had just whacked me across the chest with a hockey stick.

Reality settled in really quickly. I was now fully aware that I had a heart attack and had just died. That was also about the time fear showed up. I hadn't had a heart-to-heart (excuse the pun) with God in a long time, and I couldn't think of a better time than now. I did not want to die again, and I prayed to God, "God, please don't let me pass out again. I don't want that feeling of passing out. Please forgive me of all my sins. I'm not sure of anything specific right now, but just forgive me of all of them." I was hoping a blanket pardon was coming my way.

Upon arriving at the emergency room, the EMTs opened up the back of the ambulance to get me out, and I was immediately surrounded by the most wondrous music I'd ever heard. It wasn't like I had headphones on and it was only in my ears; it was all around. I could hear it above me, behind me - everywhere. This music was not like anything I had ever heard on Earth, and I have no words to describe it. I remember asking the EMTs and my wife, who had followed me to the hospital, if they had heard this glorious music. They looked at me like I was nuts, which was probably very true. As soon as my stretcher crossed the threshold into the emergency room, the music stopped. I guess it was back to business.

Dr. Shah is the founder of Carolina Cardiology in Rock Hill, S.C., and he met me in the E.R. He started giving orders for different types of medicines, like a clot-buster, pain medication, etc. Not much time elapsed before the pain started to ease, and I felt much better.

After a couple of hours of being stabilized, they transferred me to the intensive care unit. In 1994, Piedmont Medical Hospital, in Rock Hill, S.C., did not have a heart catheterization lab. The next day, Dr. Shah wanted to transfer me to a Charlotte hospital to have a heart catheterization done to determine which arteries were blocked. I knew this would raise insurance questions, as I was in charge of our insurance program at work. I did not want to get stuck with a $50,000 bill just because I did not get some kind of pre-approval. At work, Helen was in charge of the insurance paperwork. As it neared 5:00 p.m., I pleaded with the doctors and my wife to call Helen and make sure this would be covered. In the days of PPOs and HMOs, one could not be too safe. I was more concerned about the bill than about myself.

The ambulance ride from Rock Hill to Charlotte was a disaster. Can somebody please explain to me why they make the width of the stretcher 6" too short on both shoulders? The Flying Wallendas, the world-renowned circus act, would not have been able to balance themselves on a stretcher! At every turn, I came off that cot and looked for something to hold onto. Once I even had to grab the EMT's leg, which promptly led to a kick. By the time we got to Charlotte, I was in the throes of another heart attack.

The good news? They gave me morphine for the

pain. The bad news? We learned that I am allergic to it. Shortly after receiving my first dose, I was cussing out nurses, doctors and family members. For some, this was not a new experience. Then I vomited all over the bed, the nurse, the walls, the floor, and myself. This led to a shot of a new drug, dilaudid, which is a synthetic morphine. If I were going to be a drug addict, this would be my drug of choice. I felt really good after that!

Next came my first experience with the heart catheterization lab. I admit that I'm always a bit nervous about the first time for anything. I never know if, or how much, it is going to hurt. I don't like pain. I was sedated for this procedure, as is common practice, however I would have preferred to be completely knocked out. They inject dye into your bloodstream, slice your femoral artery near your groin, insert a catheter, and thread it into the heart. To keep you from bleeding to death while they slice the femoral artery, they stick a valve in the artery. I think they called it a shunt valve, but I was sedated so I'm not sure. The doctor watches the procedure on a monitor to determine if there are any plumbing problems (clogs) in the coronary arteries. During this procedure they can perform an angioplasty, and now they can place a stent. At the time of my procedure, stents had not been invented yet.

They determined that I had a blockage in the left anterior descending coronary artery (LAD), which flows blood to the left ventricle. They refer to this as the "widow maker," as it is usually fatal. Your left ventricle is very important because it is the main pumping chamber for your body. Your right ventricle pumps blood to your lungs, so it is smaller. If the left ventricle stops pumping, it is usually fatal. They performed a couple of angioplasties, and I was sent to recovery.

While alone in recovery, I started having convulsions. My arms and legs were flailing around like a fish out of water. I had no control over this, which was very upsetting. The whole time I thought, "I'm going to have another heart attack in the recovery room, and nobody will ever notice." After what seemed like half an hour, but was probably more like five minutes, some nurses finally noticed me flopping around and covered me with some hot blankets, which ended my convulsions. I was so happy to hear, "Art, you must be allergic to the (contrast) dye." I wanted so badly to say, "You think?"

A day or two later, I was back in the catheterization lab to have a balloon pump inserted into my heart. At the time, I didn't realize these things are only used in critical situations. They told me the pump was used to help take the workload off the heart. This meant that I had to get the other side of my groin sliced open and the balloon pump inserted up another major artery. Now both sides of my groin were sliced open with valves inserted, and my legs were immobilized with sandbags.

They kept me pretty sedated for a few days. One day my colleagues came by, perhaps to say goodbye, as things were looking pretty grim at that point. I don't remember things being all that bad; I was pretty much at peace, filled with dilaudid. I do remember, however, the beep of the heart balloon pump every second or two, and wishing they could hit the mute button.

Unfortunately, my procedures were not yet complete. A few days later, Dr. Shah came in and said he wanted to take the balloon pump out. I figured it was no big deal; it was easy in, easy out. Wrong. I had several nurses on both sides of the bed, their faces filled with concern. Now that made me wonder, "How many people does it take to pull out a balloon pump?" This thought was followed by, "What do they know that I don't?" Dr. Shah asked me several times if I was ready, to which I responded, "Sure," every time. I mean, how bad could it be? What happened next made waterboarding seem like kids' play.

As Dr. Shah looked at the nurses on each side of me and counted to three, he ripped the balloon pump out in one motion. At the same time, the nurses removed the valves on both sides of my groin in milliseconds. Then they both pushed down on each side of my groin with as much force as they could muster. My immobile legs shot straight up, and I let out a scream straight from a horror movie. I've never felt so much pressure and pain, especially in such a sensitive area.

After a few minutes, I got used to this feeling, and my legs settled back down to their original position. I made a mental note to never date a nurse, because anybody who had this kind of knowledge could not be trusted. Next, they brought in c-clamps that I swear came directly from Home Depot. They proceeded to remove their hands from my groin and clamp me down to the bed with these $5.99 clamps. This did not feel much better than the hand pressure. I remained this way for the next couple of hours. Every now and then, the nurse would release a small amount of pressure by backing off the clamp.

It took a while to figure out what this whole procedure was about. I think it would have been much easier if they would have told me from the beginning what they were doing and why. They could have said something like, "Art, we are going to remove this balloon pump and the valves from your groin. In order to keep you from bleeding to death, since we have sliced open the two largest arteries in your legs, we will have to apply direct pressure to your groin until we are sure these arteries have closed." I would have understood, and I would have been better prepared for this torture. I'm sure my heart would have appreciated that as well. Where is the truth when you need it?

There is a saying in the world of cardiology that "time is muscle." The sooner you get to a hospital and get blood flowing again to the affected area of your heart, the less muscle damage occurs. My pride increased that time by almost two hours and caused the loss of a lot of muscle in my heart. The tremendous pain I had felt was actually my heart muscle dying. I could have easily walked the few blocks to the hospital near my office and avoided most, if not all, of that damage. My pride kept me in denial, however, and I chose to go home instead. That decision had life-long consequences. My advice to you if you have even the most remote feeling of chest pain, surrender your pride and get to the hospital. Pride and denial are a deadly combination. It led to my death 15 years later on June 11, 2009.

Below are the signs of a heart attack from the American Heart Association:

CHEST DISCOMFORT:

Most heart attacks involve discomfort in the center of the chest that lasts more than a few minutes, or that goes away and comes back. It can feel like uncomfortable pressure, squeezing, fullness or pain.

DISCOMFORT IN OTHER AREAS OF YOUR BODY:

Symptoms can include pain or discomfort in one or both arms, the back, neck, jaw or stomach.

SHORTNESS OF BREATH:

With or without chest discomfort.

OTHER SIGNS:

Breaking out in a cold sweat, nausea or lightheadedness.

FOR WOMEN:

As with men, women's most common heart attack symptom is chest pain or discomfort. But women are somewhat more likely than men to experience some of the other common symptoms, particularly shortness of breath, nausea/vomiting, and back or jaw pain.

CALLING 911

Some heart attacks are sudden and intense. But most heart attacks start slowly, with mild pain or discomfort. Often people affected aren't sure what's wrong, and wait too long before getting help. Immediately call 9-1-1 so an ambulance (ideally with advanced life support) can be sent for you.

Learn the signs, but remember this: Even if you're not sure it's a heart attack, have it checked out (tell a doctor about your symptoms). Minutes matter! Fast action can save lives — maybe your own. Don't wait more than five minutes to call 9-1-1 or your emergency response number.

Calling 9-1-1 is almost always the fastest way to get lifesaving treatment. Emergency medical services (EMS) staff can begin treatment when they arrive — up to an hour sooner than if someone gets to the hospital by car. EMS staff are also trained to revive someone whose heart has stopped. Patients with chest pain who arrive by ambulance usually receive faster treatment at the hospital, too. It is best to call EMS for rapid transport to the emergency room.

For more information, visit the American Heart Association's for more information at: http://www.heart.org/HEARTORG/

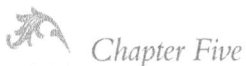
Chapter Five

PAST BEHAVIOR PREDICTS FUTURE HEALTH

After my first heart attack in 1994, I spent six months at home in rehabilitation. I asked God nearly everyday, now that He had my attention, what was next? But I still wasn't on the best of terms with God. I was telling Him what His will for my life was; I followed my own desires relating to my job, my friends, and just about everything else in my life. I figured now, though, might be the time to let Him speak. Guess what? I heard nothing. I'm not sure why God didn't open up the heavens, shout at me, or set the bush on fire. He certainly had my attention and I was all ears. Everyday I would go out and walk just a little bit farther than the day before. "God, what do you want me to do?" Nothing.

Based on that interrogation of God, I assumed I was supposed to go back to my same job, which I did. Looking back now I don't think God cared so much where I "worked" as much as His desire to have a relationship with me. Sometimes silence is an answer.

Initially, I was allowed to work part-time for a week or two, and I went back full-time after that. Shortly after my return to work, I was approached by some of the younger guys in the office to go whitewater rafting the next weekend in West Virginia on the New River. It is beyond me why they call it the New River; it is supposedly the oldest river in the world. After six months of recuperation, I figured this would be a good test of my recovery and a chance for my wife and I to have some fun together without the kids. We had been rafting numerous times while we lived in the Asheville area, and we considered ourselves just shy of expert.

We woke up early Saturday morning, ate breakfast, and made our way down to the staging area. We picked out paddles and life jackets as the guides explained the ins and outs of our all-day trip. It had been about 10 years since we had been rafting, but the safety talk seemed about the same to me. We picked out a raft that had two other couples in it and introduced ourselves. We shoved off, hoping to enjoy the wild and wonderful New River.

The morning passed quickly and without much excitement. We found a spot to picnic with other groups, and the guides made an excellent lunch for everyone. Before we shoved off again, our guide described the remaining rapids left in our trip and the approximate time to finish.

We arrived at the next-to-last rapid unscathed. Our guide asked us if we would like to beach the raft on a rock in the middle of the river and watch the other rafts go through the rapid. We all agreed that sounded like a great idea. So we paddled to the middle of the river and landed on a big rock. We watched several rafts pass by when he yelled that it was our turn. He leaned his body and paddle as far back as he could into the river. About that time, the weight of his body pushed the rear of the raft into the fast-moving river. In seconds, the right side of the raft filled up with water, forcing the left side straight up in the air. Gravity kicked in, and everybody on the left side fell into everybody on the right side. Three of us on the right side of the raft were knocked into the river.

I was immediately swept around to the other side of the rock. My safety training kicked in, and I knew I needed to get my legs pointed downriver to protect me from any rocks. The last place my legs were supposed to be was on the bottom of the river, where they could get caught on something. But the more I tried to get my legs in front of me, the more they were getting sucked straight down to the river bottom. About this time, I realized my head was underwater, and I had not taken a breath of air before going under. I figured that my life jacket would bring me to the surface, but it didn't work. I tried with all my might to force myself up out of the water to get some air. Daylight was a foot above my head, and only the river rushing over me kept me from the surface. "Life" was only a foot away, and I couldn't reach it.

I thought somebody from the raft would stick a paddle down, or throw me a rope, to pull me out.

Panic set in when I realized nobody was coming to my rescue. My lungs were screaming for air. It seemed like I had been underwater for several minutes, as everything was happening in slow motion. I looked up one last time at the top of the river and thought, "God, I can't believe I'm going to drown in this f—ing river after surviving a heart attack six months ago. We were just fooling around on that rock, and now I'm going to die. What a stupid way to die!" As soon as I reached the bottom of the river, the whirlpool that I was in dissipated. I noticed how rocky the bottom felt, and I saw a lot of limbs you could get caught on. Finally, my life jacket shot me up to the surface.

Air never felt so good, and I took the biggest breath I could. I turned around and saw that everyone in the raft looked terrified. I knew for sure they would throw me a rope immediately to pull me out of the river. Unfortunately, I was immediately sucked into another whirlpool. By then, I was completely worn out and told God, "I can't fight this anymore, so just take me wherever you want to take me." I went to the bottom of the river, and it shot me straight back up to the top. I landed on the opposite side of the river from the raft. I yelled for them to come get me, and the guide yelled back for me to swim across the river to the raft. At this point, I thought a refund was definitely due.

After a few more yelling matches and resting on the side of the river, I started to swim across the river. About halfway across, I remembered that rolling onto your back can be easier than swimming in a river. Completely exhausted at that point and questioning all my decision-making skills, I rolled onto my back and lumbered the rest of the way across the river. As I got close to the raft, the guide grabbed my life jacket and threw me into the bottom of the raft. I thought, "It's about time you did something right." I finished the last rapid in the bottom of the raft, praying I would not end up in the river again. I have not been whitewater rafting since.

Looking back now, there is a great life lesson in this adventure. When you get caught up in one of life's whirlpools, and you will, no matter how well-balanced you think your raft is, remember this. When your efforts to come up to the surface are in vain, nobody is there to save you, and you are cussing God out for the situation you are in, it's time to let go. Sometimes it is better not to try to control a situation, especially if you are in a whirlpool, and just let the river take you where it will. Before you know it, you will be back on top of the river, alive, and sucking in that wonderful air.

Held Together by Stents

Over the next four years, I was in the hospital once or twice every year for doctors to insert a stent or two to open up the blocked arteries in my heart. I became an expert. I knew it was a two-day procedure, followed by a couple of days of limited lifting and no work. For me, it didn't seem like that big of a deal, compared to completely changing my lifestyle. I didn't make any lifestyle changes at this point because the stent procedure seemed so easy.

One of the first stent procedures after my first heart attack was actually very interesting. I was in the catheterization lab, sedated, and my cardiologist had located the blockage in my coronary artery. He was getting ready to put the stent in place when all the monitors went out. He looked at the nurses and technicians and said, "Reboot." One of them replied, "We did." He responded with, "Try the F2 key." I started to laugh inwardly; this could only happen to me. I figured nobody would believe this story. I thought, "You know, that is probably not something you want to hear your cardiologist say." They decided to move me to another catheterization lab, which involved changing beds. I thought, "Watch these knuckleheads get the catheter wrapped around part of this bed, and when they lift me over to the new bed, they rip my coronary artery to shreds." Luckily for me, none of that happened.

About a year later, I was experiencing chest pain and went in for another stent or two. After the procedure, they removed the catheter and brought out the dreaded c-clamp for my groin. By now, I knew what to expect and was prepared for the hour of fun. I was in my room, minding my own business, waiting for my femoral artery to close. The nurse looked at her watch and decided to take some pressure off the clamp. What we didn't know was that when the clamp was first applied, some blood had leaked out of the site and adhered to the top of the clamp. As she backed the clamp off my groin to relieve some of the pressure, my artery opened up for no more than a split-second, and blood flew all over the room.

I was amazed at how much blood exploded out of my leg. There was blood on the bed, on the floor, on the nurse, on me - everywhere. I immediately understood how a person could die in a knife fight in a matter of seconds. The nurse tightened the clamp down, shutting off the artery, much quicker than she had opened it a few moments earlier. So a one-hour groin clamping turned into a three-hour event. The nurse was nice enough to stay in my room and keep me company until that Home Depot c-clamp was removed.

In 1999, I had been separated from my wife for

about three months when I felt chest pain, and I knew it was time to go back in for another routine stent, or so I thought. I was in my favorite catheterization lab when my cardiologist mumbled something about not being able to stent a stent. He said I needed a bypass operation immediately. Sedated, I thought, "Why not?" This really is not a decision you should make with your groin sliced open and under the influence of some really good drugs. Considering how much pain I was feeling in my chest, I said, "Sure, do whatever you've got to do."

The next thing I knew, a nurse stuck a bunch of papers under my nose, telling me I had to sign them before they could proceed. Are contracts really valid when one of the parties is drugged out of his mind? All I know is that pain will make you do some pretty crazy things.

I signed my life away, and two nurses walked in carrying electric razors. They proceeded to remove all of my sheets, which is cruel and unusual punishment. It's just not right for a man to be naked in a 45-degree room. Then they started shaving areas that God never meant to be shaved. Shortly thereafter, they dropped their electric razors and starting using shaving cream and razor blades in the aforementioned areas. There is not a drug strong enough to cover up this profound humiliation. I was scarred for life, before the surgery even started.

Fortunately, the anesthesiologist showed up and removed my consciousness from further humiliation. I woke up several hours later, however, to a new misery. It seems the recovery room experts felt it would be good for me to wake up with a tube in my throat breathing for me. A little forewarning would have been appreciated with this nightmare. When it comes to survival instincts, gagging and not being able to breathe are at the top of my list of things to fight. It is not good to wake up with overwhelming terror. I immediately tried to rip out whatever was in my throat that was keeping me from breathing. Evidently that didn't sit well with the nurses, who came out of nowhere to pin my arms down. I know I took three or four of them with me before they knocked me out again.

I woke up a few hours later without a tube in my throat, much to my immense relief. Then I noticed the bandage on my chest and the most intense pain I had felt in a long time. I spent the most miserable week of my life in the hospital. The pain medicine they gave me barely helped. On a scale of 1-10, with 10 being excruciating, I would say I stayed at about 8.5 all week. I have no idea how somebody in their 60s or 70s survives this surgery. I was 42.

My sister Beth came from Ohio to help me during my first week at home. I'm not sure how I would have survived that first week on my own, as the combination of painkillers and Xanax made me hallucinate most of the day. I was talking to the wall, and it was talking back to me.

For 42 years, I had fallen asleep on my stomach. Now I was stuck sleeping on my back. Any movement to roll over to my side was met with excruciating pain, as my chest cavity was still raw from being sliced open with a chain saw. I don't think your body was ever meant to be sliced down the middle and spread apart. It would take another four or five months to be able to sleep on my side without pain waking me up. It took a year before I could sleep on my stomach without pain. I made a promise to myself that I would never have my chest cracked open again. I would rather die than repeat that kind of suffering.

The surgeon who performed the surgery requested that I visit his office two weeks after I got home to inspect the incision and see how the skin was healing. I had to keep the bandage and the incision dry when I showered. This wasn't too hard; the first time water hit my chest, I thought I would pass out from the pain. I pretty much backed into the shower and stayed that way for a month.

When I returned to the surgeon, I took off my shirt and lay down on the examination bed. He came in and removed the bandage. He poked the scar tissue with his finger and mumbled something about not liking how the skin was healing. He said he would have to cauterize the wound again. That didn't sound good to me, and what he did next confirmed my suspicions. He asked the nurse for a scalpel and some sodium nitrate. Before I could voice any concerns, he slit my scar open and was dabbing the sodium nitrate in my wound with a Q-tip. I think I was in shock, realizing he had just sliced my chest open without using local anesthesia. He put a new bandage on the wound and said he wanted to see me in two weeks. I left muttering something about Nazi doctors.

Every day for the next two weeks I checked my wound to see how it was healing. It looked fine to me. Against my better judgment, I went back to *der doktor,* thinking he would agree. He proceeded to repeat the same scenario as the first time. However, this time I stopped him and inquired about some local anesthesia. He replied that there were no pain nerves in scar tissue, and he sliced me open again. I know - fool me once, shame on you, fool me twice, shame on me. But this was 1999, not 1899. He never got to see how the skin healed after that.

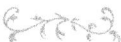

LIFE IN 10-POUND INCREMENTS

I can mark my life in ten-pound increments. I graduated high school at 155 lbs., and at 5'8" that was pretty normal. I graduated college at 165. I got married at 175. Lauren was born when I was 185. I changed jobs at 195. Matt was born when I weighed 205. I had my first heart attack at 215, which was 60 pounds heavier than my high school graduation. My marriage deteriorated along with my health. I had a triple bypass at 225. I got divorced at 230 pounds.

I was consciously committing what I now call food suicide. My thought process went something like this, "I might as well enjoy it today, because I might

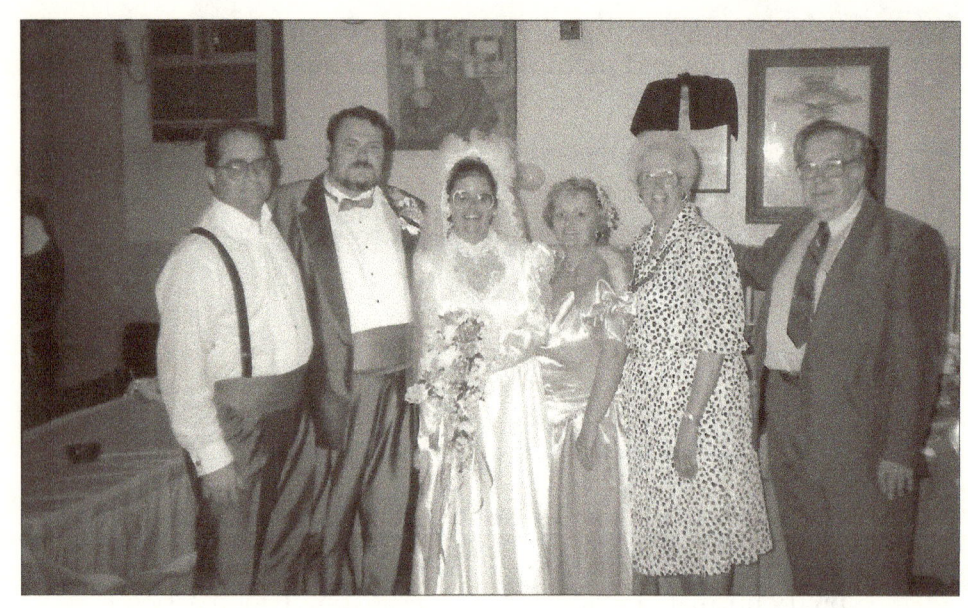

At my sister's wedding in the mid-1990's. I'm the slim one on the left.

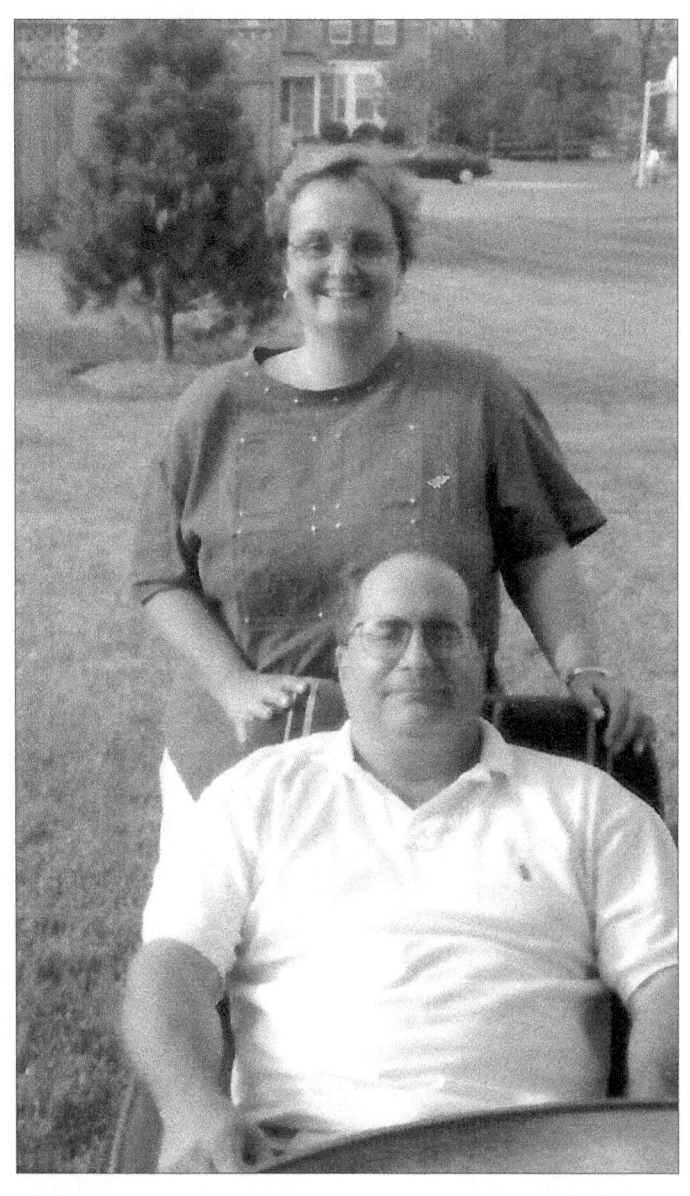

Me at my maximum weight after my divorce, 2004.

die tomorrow." I used this misguided thinking to justify eating any amount of whatever I wanted, especially when it came to hamburgers, pizza, and barbeque.

I told myself:

"I only need to live long enough to see my kids graduate high school. That's longer than my parents lived."

"Heart disease just runs in my family. There's nothing I can do about it."

I was literally eating myself to death. Food had become one of the few pleasures in my life, and despite all the warning signs I got from my heart, I couldn't stop the unhealthy eating I relied on as a comfort.

I spent the five years after my bypass being compliant with everything my cardiologist prescribed. My regimen consisted of aspirin, a cholesterol-lowering pill, a blood pressure pill, a beta-blocker, and nitroglycerin. My blood numbers improved tremendously, and I felt I had turned a corner on heart disease. My cholesterol, lipids, and triglycerides were all where they were supposed to be. I did everything I was supposed to, except change my lifestyle.

In 2004, however, I felt that familiar pain in my chest and went in for another stent. Before being discharged, I asked the cardiologist why I needed a stent after all my blood numbers had been spot-on for five years. He looked at me and said, "Art, if I were you, I'd make sure everything is right between you and your pastor." Then he walked out of my room.

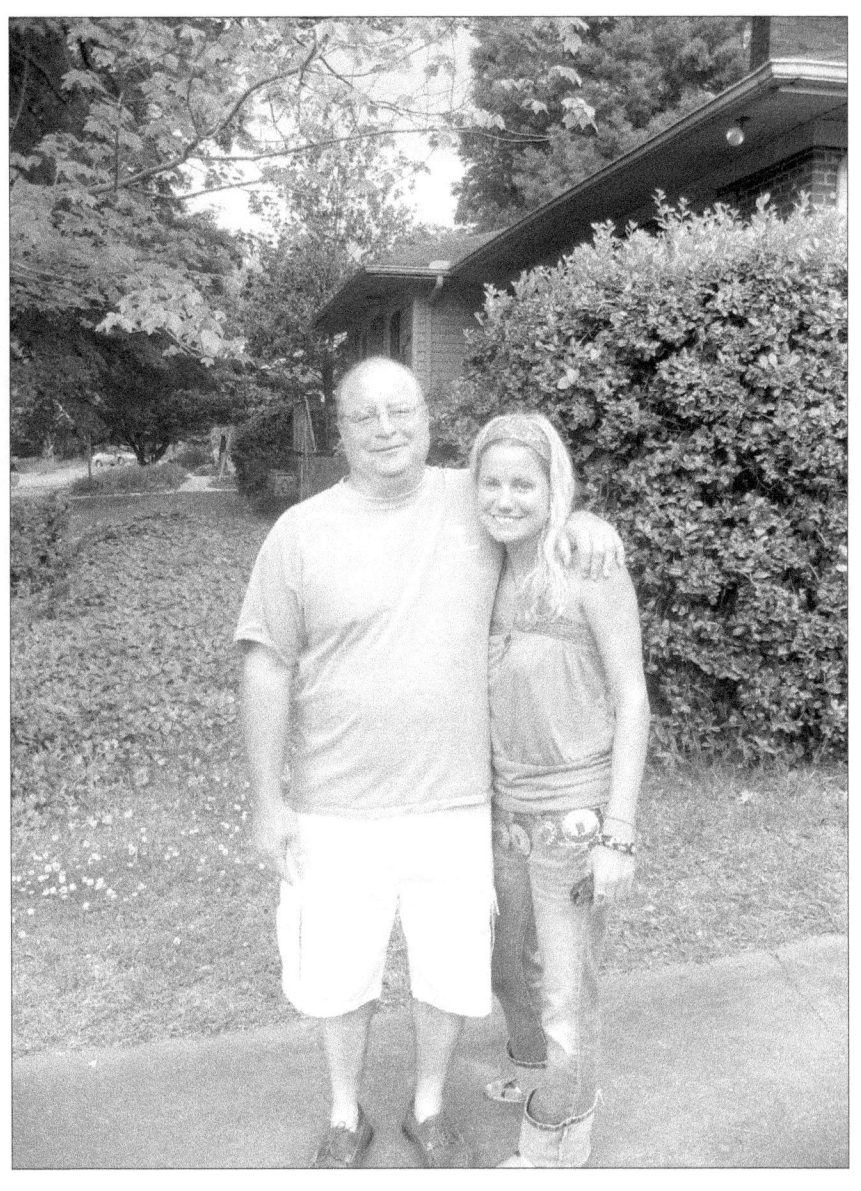

My daughter Lauren and me before my weight loss.

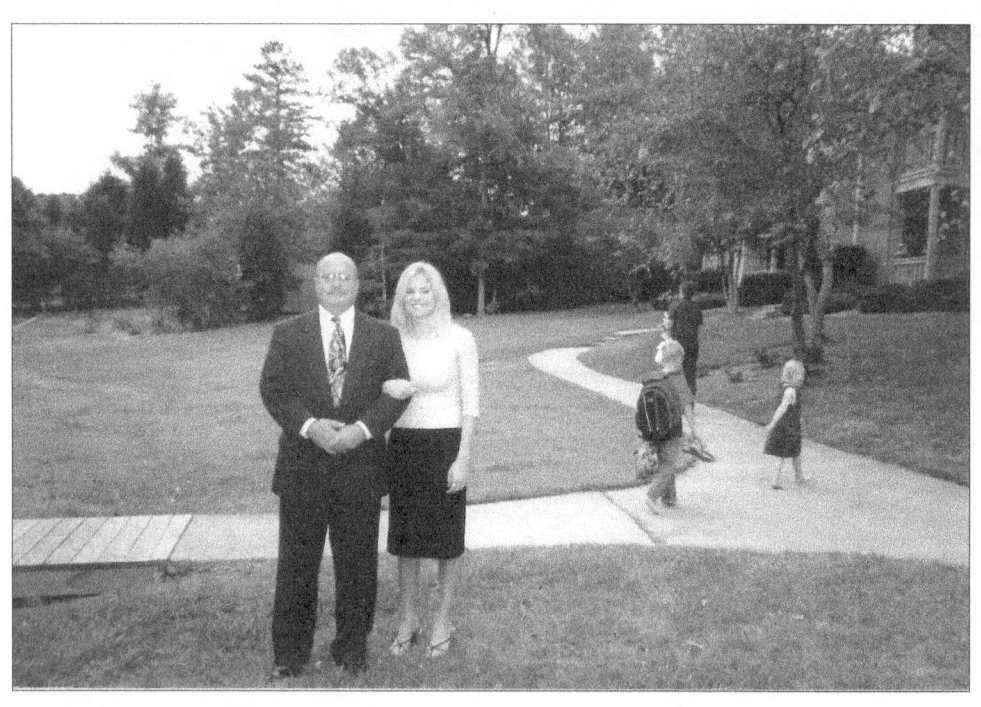

Lauren's Homecoming, Life as a Single Dad

I lay there on the hospital bed, and I became livid. I thought to myself, "All I have done for 10 years is take the medicine you prescribed, follow your instructions, and let you slice me open numerous times, and that's your answer? You have done nothing to cure this disease." I knew then that I needed to do something else.

The one thing I had never focused on during my ten-year battle with heart disease was what I was stuffing in my mouth everyday. At 47, I had myself convinced that I just could not lose weight. I was too old, and my metabolism had slowed down too much to make weight loss a possibility. However, my attitude became, "Well, what do I have to lose?" I thought I would try a more heart-friendly diet, mixed in with some heart-healthy vitamins, minerals, and oils. I started dating a woman who was fanatical about eating and weight control. She read Dr. Dean Ornish's book on reversing heart disease. She made a plan for me that was pretty simple, and, with a little discipline, it worked for me. The plan was to limit fat to 25 grams a day, limit portion size, and walk 30 minutes a day several times a week. The weight came off slowly. I would lose one pound a week, or maybe two pounds on a good week. Over the course of the next year, I dropped 5-6 pounds a month. That may not sound like much, but it added up to 65 pounds at the end of the year. I went from 230 pounds to 165.

One of the most critical aspects of my weight loss was portion control. I had never disciplined myself with portion control, unless it was something I didn't like.

If I liked something, I would eat it until I felt stuffed, which was usually 3,000 calories later. Portion control is a lot easier if you can address the most important aspect of eating; I call it your emotional connection to food. Most, if not all, diets fail for this reason. They never address the emotional reasons for eating. Eating makes us feel better. We eat to reward ourselves. We look at food as comfort. We eat because we are mad and deserve that gallon of ice cream. We eat because we had a tough day at the office. We eat because we just had a fight with our spouse. The list goes on and on. You may have heard the saying, "eat to live or live to eat." Well, it's true! So few of us eat to live. If we would view food as merely fuel for our bodies, America would be a whole lot healthier. Until you identify and understand your emotional connection to food and break that connection, food will always be a problem. Breaking the emotional connection to food for me was easy. The emotional connection I had with food was transferred to being in an emotional relationship. For you it might be a hobby or sport, personal time alone, reading, watching a movie, or spending time with the opposite sex.

Losing weight is simple, but it's not easy until you break that emotional connection. It's simple because it's simple math. A pound of fat is 3,500 calories. If you reduce just 500 calories a day out of your life, that adds up to 3,500 calories a week. Losing one pound a week, every week for a year, is a loss of 52 pounds. You

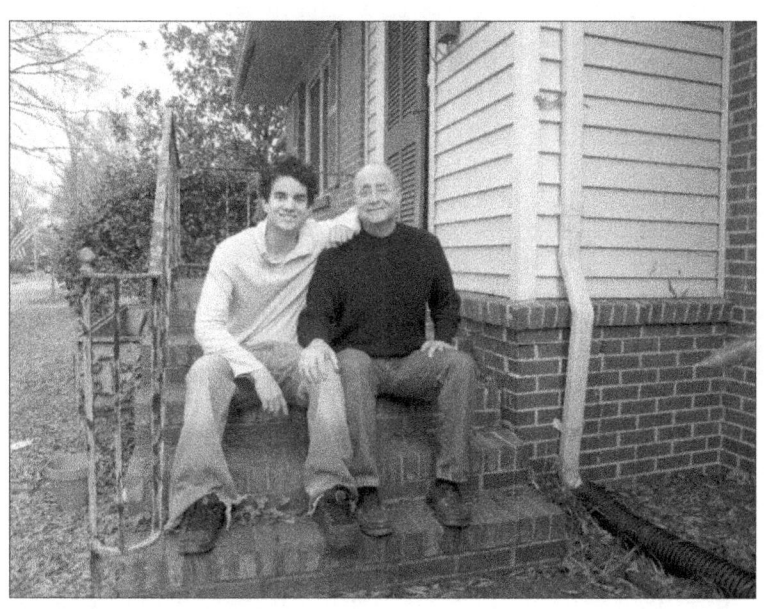

My youngest son Matt and I after my weight loss.

don't need to be Einstein to understand this. If I could do this at 47, anybody can.

It felt so great to buy smaller jeans every couple of months. I went from a size 40 waist to a 32. I went from wearing XL shirts to wearing mediums. I realized my body image had had a negative impact on my self-image. I felt so much better about myself at 165 pounds, and I knew my heart appreciated it as well. I also loved hearing from people I hadn't seen in a while how good I looked. I always loved that saying, "That cookie doesn't taste as good as a size 6 feels."

I want you to know that losing weight doesn't necessarily mean you are now healthy. This is a big misconception that cost me my life. I lost 65 pounds, and a few years later I was lying dead at the YMCA. You can lose weight just by practicing portion control and cutting in half all the junk that you are currently eating. However, if you don't replace that junk with healthy, nutritious food, your arteries are still susceptible to clogging and you will not be healthy. I will talk about this more in Chapter 10.

My relationship with Ms. Nutrition lasted about 18 months. Although things didn't work out romantically, I decided to look at the positive things that came as a result. She had gotten me to lose 65 pounds, and I felt great about myself for the first time in a long time. You have to be grateful for the people God places in your life, no matter the length of time they are there. Just know there is a reason God has placed them there. You might need to learn a lesson, or they might meet a need in your life. They might also help you grow, or you might even teach them something. Just don't ignore them or take them for granted.

For the next five years, 2004 to 2009, I did not darken the door of a doctor. I was walking a couple of miles most days, practicing portion control the majority of the time, and keeping my weight between 165 and 170. I felt great, and my heart felt great. I saw no reason to see a doctor and start taking a bunch of medicine again.

In May of 2009, however, I became short of breath while working out at the YMCA. I was also having difficulty breathing while lying down and sleeping at night. Then, I gained ten pounds in one week, even though my eating habits had not changed. At that point, I figured it was time to go see my cardiologist. He did several tests, and a week later he called me in to tell me I had congestive heart failure.

I don't think my decision to take a sabbatical from the medical community contributed to my congestive heart failure. It had been 15 years since my first heart attack, which had done the initial damage to my left ventricle. The muscle that dies during a heart attack develops scar tissue and makes contractions harder for the heart. To compensate for this, the heart becomes enlarged over time as it tries to keep up with the body's demand for blood.

An enlarged heart eventually becomes weaker and weaker. Instead of ejecting the normal 60-65% of the blood entering the left ventricle, it ejects half of that or less. My ejection fraction was 12%. I never knew about this process until last year. That is why it is so critical to get to the hospital when you feel chest pain. The sooner those arteries can be opened up and blood flow restored to the affected heart muscle, the less chance of any muscle tissue dying. I could have avoided all of this if I had simply gone down the block to the hospital that day when I was 37 and got my arteries opened immediately. But I lied to myself and said that it was just indigestion. This is what pride will do to you. Guys, just lay your man card down and get to the hospital.

The doctor prescribed some blood pressure medicine and a diuretic to remove the fluid build-up in my body. The diuretic worked great. I lost those ten pounds in a couple of days and went right back to my normal life.

I never knew that congestive heart failure could lead to cardiac arrest. Evidently, the scar tissue on the left ventricle can disrupt the electrical system, causing your heart to have a life-threatening arrhythmia. Wouldn't you think that would come under the full disclosure principle? I would have liked that information before I headed out to the YMCA to work out that night.

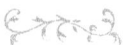

I firmly believe that 80-90% of Americans could avoid this disease with a few lifestyle changes. Fat, salt, and sugar are killing America. If you want to change your life, change what and how much you eat. Show me your meals, and I'll show you your future. Don't trade short-term pleasure for long-term pain. I tried it, and it doesn't work.

Chapter Six

YOU CALL THIS RECOVERY?

Near the end of June in 2009, I was released from the hospital. My ICD that I had debated having implanted had been safely put in a couple of days before my release, and I was really looking forward to going home and sleeping in my own bed. As the nurse went over the discharge instructions and asked for my signature, I was much more focused on getting out of there. For all I knew, I could have signed anything that morning.

Despite my desire to get home, I was a little apprehensive about leaving the hospital. There is some comfort knowing if something happens, you are right there for immediate attention. I also had no confidence in this piece of machinery implanted in my chest. Given my history with mechanical malfunctions, I was half-expecting this thing to shock me every time a pretty woman walked by. They told me "if" I did get shocked, it would feel like getting kicked in the chest by a horse. Little did I know, "if" would turn into "when." I sarcastically thought, "Great, I can't wait to experience that. I just love horses. Not."

But I did remind myself that I was only a mile away from the hospital.

My youngest son, Matt, drove me home. It was strange not having been home for nearly three weeks. As I walked into my house, everything just felt different. It was a weird feeling. Having lived by myself for a couple of years, I had come to know where I put most things, except my car keys. Perhaps things were in different places now. I now understood how Papa Bear felt about Goldilocks. I was finally home, though, and it felt good. Matt ran to the store to get some groceries. Upon his return, I jumped up out of my chair to help him bring in the groceries, and I immediately passed out.

I woke up to hear Matt talking to the 911 operator, saying, "My dad just came home from the hospital, and he collapsed." Hearing this from the middle of floor, I thought, "I just got home; I can't go back to the hospital. I haven't been home an hour, and I'm not going back to the hospital. I'm really OK." I looked at Matt and told him several times, "I'm OK, I'm OK. I just stood up too fast." Thankfully, he hung up and ordered me to sit while he put away the groceries. I figured now might be a good time to read those discharge instructions. I guess they were serious about the getting up slowly part.

I couldn't wait to sleep in my own bed that night. I turned the light out, and everything that had happened to me since June 11 came to mind. I felt like the luckiest man alive to have a second, or more like a fifth or six, chance at life. I tried to fall asleep, but the "what if" questions started to bombard my brain. "Where's my faith now?" I wondered. Since I had had an arrhythmia in the middle of the night, just a few nights ago, I was afraid of another one. Every time I moved, I wondered if it would set off the ICD. Since it was so new in my body, I wasn't used to it. What would happen if one of the leads going into my heart broke off?

Then there was the fear of death. Was I ready to die? I knew I would go to heaven, but was I really ready to leave this world? The hardest part was that it wasn't an event 10 or 20 years in the future. It was staring me in the face right then. I simply was not ready to die. I had unspoken words to say to family, friends, etc. I had places to visit, grandkids to watch grow up, and the list went on. I wanted to live. I wanted to love and be loved. Then I realized it wasn't my will, but rather it was God's will. It was really up to God if I would be given another day.

I woke up in the middle of night with night sweats. My head and pillow were soaked. I thought, "You better get a hold of yourself, or they will be sticking you back in the hospital!" This went on for the next three or four nights, and then it stopped just as quickly as it started. I figured my subconscious mind eventually got used to the piece of metal in my chest, and my conscious mind trusted it a little more each day.

July was pretty uneventful. Matt eventually had to go back to work in Lexington, SC, after missing nearly a month between June and July. He had made a huge sacrifice to stay with me. I was not allowed to drive for three months, due to the electrical issues in my heart. That meant I had to rely on friends or family for every trip I wanted to take. To get around, I was totally dependent on others. I had been independent for so long that asking others for help felt completely unnatural to me. It was the hardest and most frustrating aspect of my recovery. I really could not accept it until one day my sister, Beth, called and told me, "Art, you have to let people help you! It's just as good for them as it is for you."

It is amazing how good people really are. The outpouring of prayers and support, as well as help with everyday tasks, was overwhelming. I really had no idea how much people cared about me. I can't tell you how many times people dropped what they were doing to take me to a doctor's appointment, the bank, or the grocery store. My neighbor not only mowed his grass, but he mowed my yard, too! That whole summer, somebody other than me did my yard work. I felt glad about that, but I also felt guilty at the same time. It was hard for me to watch somebody else do what I normally could have done.

One day I was being driven to lunch, and a question

entered my mind. As we exited the interstate, I asked God, "Why didn't you bring me back to life after three or four shocks? Why 16 shocks, God?" His response was, "I could have brought you back to life after three or four shocks, but who would have received the glory for that?" I thought, "Man would have." He said, "After 16 shocks, is there any doubt who should receive the glory?" I couldn't argue that one with Him.

I expected my recovery to go like all the prior ones. I figured each day I would get a little better and in a couple of weeks, I would be back to normal. Wrong. I was not bouncing back like I thought I would. I had one or two good days, and then I would have a couple of bad days. One day I was completely tired, and I felt great the next. Between the lack of independence and the ups and downs of my recovery, it would have been easy to get depressed. But I decided to focus on the fact that I was still alive, and I tried to remember that God must have a reason for me being here.

I took that attitude into the month of August. The doctor said when it came to exercise, I should do as much as I could, but I should listen to my body. I began a short walking routine and tried to increase it daily, but I didn't have much success. I'd get maybe 500 yards or so from my house, start to feel something funny in my chest, and I would have to go home. One night, I decided to walk my dog. We made it about two houses when I had the distinct feeling that I was passing out. I immediately sat down on the curb. I waited several minutes and got up to go home. I walked about 10 feet and had the same sensation again, so I sat down again. This repeated itself a few more times until I was sitting directly across from my house. I was only about 100 feet from my house, sitting on the curb and contemplating the possibility of crawling to the front door. I knew if I could get home and lie on my bed, this would all pass.

I'm not one to call the doctor every time my nose runs, but I figured they might want to know about this little incident. In the morning, I called the doctor's office and left a message. A little bit later, they called back and asked what happened the night before. They suggested I walk the dog early in the day when it wasn't so hot. That sounded good to me. It was about lunchtime when we ventured out, when the temperature was in the 70s as opposed to the high 90s.

I figured it was as good a time as ever to test their theory. I lassoed up my wild and uncontrollable lab pup and headed out for a walk. I was paying particular attention to my heart; I knew at the first sign of getting lightheaded I would find a curb to sit down on. At the end of my street, about a ½ mile from the house, I got lightheaded, so I looked at the curb and told myself to sit down.

My world immediately went black. When my eyes opened again, all I could see was this concrete curb coming up to my face very quickly. I had no time to put out my hands to break my fall, and the only thought that raced through my mind was, "God, this is going to hurt." Just about that time, I face-planted into the curb full-force. I hit the curb and thought, "God, that <u>did</u> hurt!" As blood poured out from different areas of my head, my loyal pup was right there, trying to lick it all up. I knew I had to get him away from the damage, so I told him to sit, which he partially did.

I took an inventory of what was hurt. I took my shirt off to figure out where I was bleeding. Blood was gushing out of my forehead and nose. My glasses were shattered, but there was no damage to my eyes. I checked my teeth, and they were all there. At that point, I had three thoughts. One, hopefully one of my neighbors was outside and saw me fall. Two, there is no way I'm going to be able to walk home from here. Three, "This is going to be another trip to the hospital. I hate stitches."

Without my glasses, I couldn't see if there were any neighbors outside. Since nobody came running up immediately, I decided to call somebody. With one hand holding my shirt up to my forehead and one hand holding the dog leash, I ran out of hands to hold my iPhone. I chose to hold the dog, so I dropped the shirt and attempted to dial. This led to another complication. Every time I dropped my shirt to dial, blood would get all over the face of my phone, which really screwed up the touch screen. To deal with this, I wiped the face clean on my jeans and attempted to make a call, all while holding onto the dog, the shirt, and the phone at the same time.

My first phone call got no answer. This meant I had to go through the same routine again. I wiped the screen clean, held the dog, the shirt, and the phone, and hoped somebody would pick up this time. I got through to my good friend Chuck, whose wife Laurie worked just a couple of miles away. I told him I was at the end of my street. He said it was no problem and that he was on it. I waited for what I thought was an appropriate amount of time for his wife to arrive before I called him back. He said Laurie was at the entrance of my street and didn't see me. "No, I said the end of the street," I told Chuck. Given the current condition of my iPhone, maybe "end" and "entrance" sounded the same.

Laurie showed up, took me and my dog home, and cleaned up my face. By now it must have looked like a Halloween mask. Then we headed to the emergency room. I looked at myself in the mirror before we left, and it only confirmed what I already knew – I needed stitches. It made me sick to my stomach to think about numbing the wound and stitching it up. I didn't mind the throbbing headache I had, but the thought of a needle going into those cuts made me woozy.

By now, I must have been on a first-name basis with the folks in the ER. It was the only time I have gone to the ER, without an ambulance, and didn't wait at all in the waiting room. They immediately rushed me into a room and began their normal procedures. The ER doctor assessed the situation and, since I had hit my head, he wanted to do a CT scan. I had been told that a CT scan has about 600 times the amount of radiation as an x-ray. I had already had about 10 CT

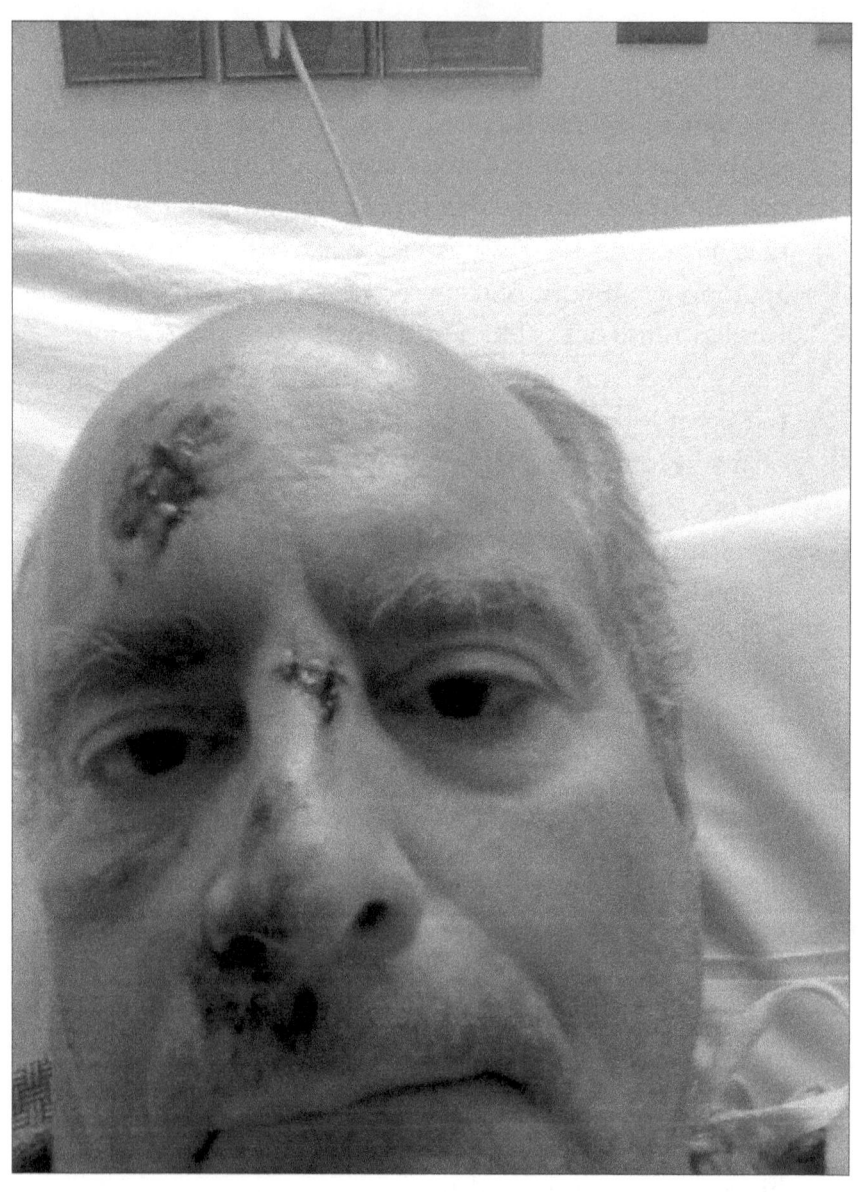

After I Hit the Curb, August 2009

scans of my head back in June when I had the strokes and blood clots. By now, I was wondering about the limit for CT scans in a year.

The results came back surprisingly quickly. The ER doctor came in with his dreaded suture kit and told me I had a slight skull fracture, broken nose, and a small air pocket behind my eye socket. The air pocket concerned them; it might lead to brain fluid loss, and they didn't want me to lay flat for the next four days.

Before the stitching started, another doctor showed up. Without my glasses, I could only see clearly about two feet in front of my face. He introduced himself as Dr. Ramos and said he had worked on me in the ER back in June. I couldn't believe it. I had been trying to track him down for a month. I had called his office several times to set up an appointment to tell him thanks, but I never got a call back. I guess an emergency room doctor doesn't keep office hours for appointments. Besides, who else would ever contact an emergency room doctor? Apparently, he saw my name on the computer screen and wanted to come by to see what was happening. I looked at him and said, "I just wanted to make sure you guys hadn't forgotten about me." He chuckled and said, "Forget about you, Art? You are a legend around here. We talk about you every day and the fact that you actually walked out of here."

He then asked if I had been calling his office and wondered why. I told him, "Yes, I just wanted to tell you thanks for saving my life!" He replied, "You don't need to thank me." I looked at him quizzically and said,

"Oh, yes I do! I really want to thank you for saving my life back in June." What he told me next just stunned me. He said, "Art, I have been doing this job for 20 years. You are the fourth person in 20 years to ever thank me. He then said that those four people were a 16-year-old pregnant girl that bled out, two heart attack patients, and myself. I looked at him in disbelief and said, "No way! You must get thanked every day or at least once a week." He responded, "Art, people either complain or cuss me out." I couldn't believe that a guy who dedicated his life to fixing people up, saving lives, setting broken bones, etc., received such little appreciation and gratitude. I immediately made a mental note to say, "Thank you," a lot more often while I was in the hospital. How sad!

He then asked if he could do anything or if I had any other questions. I said, "Just one more question. I want to know what made you shock me 11 times. Why didn't you stop after three or four or eight times?" He laughed and said, "It could have been more than 11 times - I lost count. But you have to know something about me. I come from a family of five boys, and we never quit at anything. Every time I shocked you, you responded. I just made up my mind that as long as you responded, I was going to keep shocking you!" I looked at him and said the first words that came to my mind, "I am so glad you're not a quitter!"

"Art, you had a whole team working on you that night. I was just calling the shots." I told him, "As a quarterback, Doc, you called all the right plays! Please tell the rest of your team I said thank you!" He smiled and resumed his ER duties. After he left, the stitching began. Around the same time, both my cardiologist and ICD rep from Biotronik arrived.

The ICD is a remarkable piece of technology. It monitors every heartbeat and rhythm. It determines immediately if there is an abnormal rhythm and if any therapy is needed. It is also programmable through the use of an external laptop. The settings can be adjusted as needed. You can also download a complete history of your heart function, from the day it was implanted or the date of the last download. This is called "interrogating the device." The ICD also communicates wirelessly every night to the Biotronik headquarters, which monitors and reports any "events" to the cardiologist's office. It does this by magic, I think.

Ben from Biotronik hooked up his laptop to my ICD via a magnetic mouse (magic again) and downloaded my information. He told me that I had two "VTs" the night before while walking my dog, and the ICD had delivered therapy. A VT is short for a ventricular tachycardia, which is a form of a cardiac arrhythmia. Ben also said that at 12:18 p.m. that day I had a VT that lasted eight seconds, and the ICD delivered therapy to get my heart back into a normal rhythm.

An arrhythmia is simply an abnormal heart rhythm. It's usually an extremely fast heartbeat. Some arrhythmias are not life-threatening and aren't that serious. These usually happen in the upper part of the heart. Other arrhythmias are life-threatening emergencies that can lead to cardiac arrest and sudden death. Unfortunately, mine fell into the second category. A VT is an arrhythmia in the lower part of your heart, better known as the ventricle. The problem with VT is that it could lead to ventricular fibrillation, which means there is an uncoordinated contraction of the ventricle, and instead of pumping blood, it just sits there and quivers. From personal experience, this is not good.

Dr. Patel, my cardiologist, looked at the downloaded information and said they needed to fine-tune the ICD. They needed to accelerate the "therapy" treatment provided by the ICD so that I would get shocked sooner, instead of passing out and face-planting into the concrete. To me, that seemed like the lesser of two evils. I could get kicked in the chest by a horse, or I could kiss the concrete with my head. I hoped we could just eliminate the arrhythmias instead.

The ICD has different therapies that it delivers to the heart via two or three leads that are implanted in different areas of the heart. Usually one lead is in the upper part of the heart, and another lead is in the bottom part. Sometimes it delivers "pacing therapy" when it recognizes an abnormal rhythm, sending a small amount of electricity to the heart to get it back on track. This therapy is not painful, and you don't notice it at all. If the ICD can't get the heart back in a normal rhythm and detects a serious arrhythmia like VT, it will charge up and "shock" the heart. It will continue doing this until either the heart gets back in rhythm, the battery runs out of power, or somebody puts a magnet over the ICD, effectively turning it off. This little machine also acts as a pacemaker and will keep your heartbeat within a predetermined range, like between 60 and 120 beats per minute. For $30,000, can you really beat this technology?

Dr. Patel came into the room to explain all this and said that he wanted to admit me to the hospital. I really wanted to go home, as it seemed like I had just gotten out of the hospital. Dr. Patel explained that he wanted to watch my heart rhythms over the weekend, and this accident I just had could have been a lot worse. I said, "OK. Admit me."

I went to the monitoring floor. This floor has monitors at the nurses' desk, in your room, and numerous places in the hall. All of them monitor the patients' heart rhythms. My good friend, Billy Evans, came by the next day to visit. After a few minutes of conversation, I suggested we go for a little walk. We got all the contraptions, cords, IV lines, and monitors situated, and we went out into the hall. As I exited the room, I looked up at one of the monitors that had all the patients on it, pointed it out to Billy and said, "Patient #22 has a really weird rhythm." As we walked down the hall past the nurses' station, the nurses started yelling, "Where's Mr. Townsend? He's not in his room!" I looked at Billy and wondered what the problem was. They found me pretty quickly and ordered me back to my room.

Evidently, I was Patient #22, and I was having an arrhythmia.

I crawled back into bed, and at first I didn't really feel that bad. I tried to focus on relaxing, but the commotion in the room made that difficult. I was more upset at the thought of the ICD going off and shocking me than anything else that was happening. I wondered how fine-tuned they had this ICD. I kept waiting for this horse to show up and kick me. I knew my ICD was going to take things into its own hands and let me have it. But it didn't, and after about 20 minutes my heart settled down.

I continued to have some erratic rhythms throughout the weekend, which led Dr. Patel to schedule another heart catheterization for Monday. I reminded him that I was allergic to the dye they used, and I had to have a day's worth of prednisone prior to the procedure. Dr. Patel then remarked about how different I was, compared to all his other patients. He said that most of his patients usually feared or disliked any procedure he recommended, and it seemed to him that I welcomed them. I just figured the better my attitude was, the quicker I would heal.

On Tuesday, Dr. Patel did the heart catheterization and came into my room with the results. He said everything was open, and although two of my bypass arteries had closed up, my heart had created two collateral arteries on its own. Isn't it amazing what the heart can do? Due to the electrical issues surrounding my heart, however, Dr. Patel suggested that I go to a more specialized heart clinic. He could transfer me to Duke, Chapel Hill, Baptist Hospital in Winston-Salem, or the

Sanger Clinic in Charlotte. I chose the Sanger Clinic in Charlotte, as it had an excellent reputation and was right down the road.

Dr. Patel said he had a good relationship with one of the doctors there, Dr. Gulati, and he would set up the transfer. It took a couple of days to get that worked out, so I patiently waited in the hospital. Finally, a week after checking into the hospital, my transfer was in progress. I asked the nurse if I could put my request in for a helicopter ride to Charlotte. I'd met my deductible, so why not? She failed to see the humor in my logic. I put the same request in with the EMTs who showed up later afternoon to transfer me. They said that they would be faster than a helicopter, so naturally I had to bet them. As soon as we were loaded up, I started my watch. I must say that I have never gotten to Charlotte that fast from Rock Hill. We were at the Carolinas Medical Center (CMC) in 23 minutes.

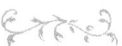

THE SANGER CLINIC

During my visit to the hospital in June, several people tried to get me transferred from Piedmont Medical Center in Rock Hill to the Sanger Clinic in Charlotte. This created some drama at the time. I understood that they had the best intentions at heart, because the Sanger Clinic does have a well-deserved, excellent reputation.

I didn't have a problem with visiting The Sanger clinic; I just didn't want to go there right then. I wasn't in any shape to be transferred; I was also dealing with more issues than just those involving my heart. At one time, I had nine doctors handling my case, and they all had to sign off on anything that any one of them wanted to do. In August, we were just dealing with a heart issue, and I gladly accepted the transfer to the Sanger Clinic.

I thought it would be a day before any doctor showed up to see me, but I was wrong. In the hours after my arrival, several Sanger doctors and nurses visited me. Each doctor had his own specialty, and I struggled to keep them straight. I also had to repeat the same story over and over. I was impressed, however, with all the attention and concern they showed. My initial impression was how they seemed to be treating my condition very aggressively. They immediately scheduled various tests.

One of these tests involved slicing my jugular vein and inserting a tube into my heart to monitor the pressure inside my heart. The nurse explained that the procedure was similar to a heart catheterization; it just used a different vein. Even I, Mr. Happy-Go-Lucky, had some trepidation about getting my neck sliced open.

They wheeled me down to the pre-operative area, which was basically a holding pattern until one of the operating rooms or catheterization labs opened up. I asked the nurse several times if they were going to give me a sedative, like they do during a heart catheterization.

She assured me every time that they would. I might as well be as relaxed as possible with a new procedure like this.

It eventually was my turn in the catheterization lab, and they commenced with all their pre-operative procedures. I still did not see anything going into my IV, so I asked again about that sedative. The nurse responded that as soon as the doctor got into the room, they would give me something. The doctor showed up and started to work on my jugular vein; I stared at my IV, and nothing was going in it. Then the doctor said that he was done. I looked at the nurse and again asked about the sedative. She responded, "Well, this procedure is so fast, we don't give the patient anything." If it hadn't been for the tube stitched into my jugular vein going into my heart, I might have lost my cool with her. I thought to myself, "This is how our relationship is going to start out? With a lie?"

Prior to moving me out of the operating room, the tube sticking out of my neck was wound up two or three times and duct-taped to my neck. Maybe it wasn't duct tape, but it sure did feel like it. I guess they needed some slack on the tubing outside of my neck. I spent the next couple of days in the intensive care unit (ICU). Evidently, to measure the pressure accurately, the bed had to be perfectly level, along with the patient. I could move some, but with this tube wrapped around my neck, I couldn't move my head to the right at all. The great thing about being in the ICU is you get a lot of personal attention. You just push a button, and somebody shows up. I wish there was an ICU button in the real world. Need money? Push a button. Hungry? Push a button. Need love? Push a button.

I guess whatever they were monitoring in my heart must have been OK; a couple of days later the nurse removed the tube from my neck. It felt great to be able to turn my neck to the right. It also meant that I was being shipped out of ICU and back to a regular bed. I underwent more basic procedures, like CT scans and x-rays, without much feedback.

By now, it was the week of August 17, and I had spent nearly two weeks in the hospital. Dr. Gulati walked in, followed by a nurse, early one morning and sat on my bed. I figured it must be something good if I was with a doctor and a nurse at the same time. Little did I know, he was about to turn my world upside down. He looked at me and said, "Art, when we consider somebody for the transplant list, we have to look at the seriousness of their life-or-death situation. You have already died once on us, and you face-planted into the concrete. Your electrical system is so bad that the best cure is for you to have a heart transplant. We could do an ablation procedure to try to limit the electrical problems, but there is so much electricity in your heart, any chance of success is minimal. Art, I know you have an ICD, but it is not infallible. I have lost patients who had ICDs, and it didn't save them. Your best bet is a transplant."

He then introduced me to his transplant coordinator, Katie, who had come in with him.

I was shell-shocked, to say the least. My mind was racing with a thousand thoughts and questions, most of them not pleasant. "A heart transplant? Are you kidding me? This is the Sanger Clinic; don't you have about 30 more tests or procedures to do before you rip my heart out? Three months ago, I thought I was healthy, and now I need a new heart?" It was too much to comprehend. I thought, "This is not happening, is it? I am only 51; I am too young for a transplant. Surely there is something else they can try!" My mind had a very difficult time wrapping itself around the idea of a transplant.

Katie launched into all the requirements, procedures, and processes involved with a heart transplant. I tried to pay attention, but my mind was in a hundred different places. I knew she was speaking, and I knew it was important, but it was going in one ear and out the other. It was reality, but I still hoped this was all just a bad dream.

Out of denial, my sense of humor returned first. Katie was so professional - actually too professional. She was so serious about all of this, which I guess is normal. For me, if we were going to have this heart transplant relationship, we should at least enjoy the process. It's *only* a matter of life and death, and I've been through this situation a few times. In her line of work, having a relationship with patients who might die could be difficult. But I now know the only things we take out of this world are love and relationships. Everything else is just "stuff."

I was now entering a new phase of my life – being a heart transplant candidate. The thought of surrendering such a vital part of my body was terrifying.

Chapter Seven

IMPLANT + FACEPLANT = TRANSPLANT

Elisabeth Kubler-Ross studied and defined the stages of grieving many years ago. They are:
- Denial
- Anger
- Bargaining
- Depression
- Acceptance

When I found out I needed a heart transplant, I passed through the first four stages of the grieving process relatively quickly. I was in **denial** for about a day. The word "transplant" was the furthest thing from my mind. It had always seemed like the last resort, and I just knew there had to be more options to explore before slicing me open again. The only **anger** I felt was directed at myself. I only had myself to blame for the shape I was in. As hard as I tried, I couldn't think of a single time anybody had held a gun to my head and made me eat that wonderfully delicious cheeseburger or pizza. I came to the conclusion that this was basically a lifestyle disease. The electrical issues in my heart were most likely caused by the scar tissue in the left ventricle, which in turn was the result of my first heart attack in 1994. The congestive heart failure was the result of an enlarged heart, which was also caused by the scar tissue. Since scar tissue in the heart doesn't do any work, the heart enlarges itself over time to compensate for the dead muscle. Had I gone to the hospital down the street to have that artery opened in 1994, there would be no dead muscle, scar tissue, electrical issues, or congestive heart failure.

Bargaining really wasn't much of an issue with me, since I didn't have anybody or anything to bargain with. If there was a do-over button in life, I would have loved to punch it. **Depression** showed up in full force that first night, which I'll talk about shortly. That leaves **acceptance**. Acceptance has not been achieved, even as I write this book 19 months later. If the transplant team ever called to say, "We have a heart for you," I would tell them to give it to somebody else. So although I think I have accepted all the information, processes, and procedures involved with a transplant, actually going through it is another matter. Right now, I just want to ride the horse I am already on as far as it will go.

Getting on the transplant list is no small feat. You are checked out from head to toe; before you get approved for a new heart, they want to make sure the rest of your body is healthy. Once the insurance company approved the initial testing, my room became the center of activity. The first nurse said she needed to get some "arterial" blood, and I didn't think anything of it. Then she added that to get arterial blood, she would need an artery. I still didn't think it was a big deal, and they could just use the same one they've been sticking for two weeks. Finally, she said, "No, to stick an artery I have to go a little deeper." This got my attention. I asked why she needed arterial blood to begin with. She responded that she needed to get an accurate oxygen count. "Whoa, whoa, whoa," I said. "That thing on my finger gives an oxygen count." I thought I had her there, and I could avoid this arterial stick. She looked at me, smiled, and replied, "Yeah but we need an *accurate* count." I was dumbfounded; why measure with this annoying little finger clamp if it's not accurate? She wiped my wrist down with alcohol and pulled out a very long needle. She stuck that thing in my wrist so far, I'm surprised it didn't come out the other side. She started to dig around for an artery, which was just a delightful feeling. I was about to give her a Google map of my arteries when her syringe started to fill up with blood.

She left, but she was immediately followed by another nurse with 18 empty vials for blood. I was just about to pass out, and I pleaded with her that I was all out of arterial blood. She smiled and said, "All I need is regular blood." I looked at the empty vials and asked, "Do you really need *that* much blood?" She responded, "Yes, we have a lot of tests to run on you." I figured at this rate I would be down two quarts by the end of the day. I would need a transfusion, not a transplant.

After she left, I went through CT scans, ultrasounds, and x-rays of all the major organs in my body. They also checked the major arteries in my neck and legs. Then they informed me that, upon my release, I would need to get copies of my dental records, eye exams, physicals, and colonoscopies. Last but not least, I would need to get a hepatitis vaccine, flu vaccine…and a partridge in a pear tree.

That night, when I was alone in my room, **depression** hit me. I figured now was as good a time as any to have a pity party. I cried for a couple of hours. I thought about all the stupid decisions I had made up to this point in my life. I thought about my pride during my first heart attack, which had caused all this damage, and how many hospitals I had driven past on the way home that day. I thought about all the junk I had shoved in my mouth over the years. I thought about my years of food suicide and how much I wanted to live now. I thought about all the pain and worry I had caused my family and friends. I thought about dying.

I cried to God through the whole thing. When I was done with my pity party, God spoke so clearly to me, "Art, I put somebody in your life before this disease began, and he was there to show you how to beat this disease. You ignored him, and you made fun of him. You were ungrateful for what he did for you. You had this entitled attitude, as if you were owed something. You ignored the very person I put in your life to help avoid all of this. His name is Lat Purser. You need to write him and ask for forgiveness."

I knew immediately He was right, and I had made a huge mistake. I worked for Lat for eleven years, from 1988-1999, and I had observed his daily ritual. He would occasionally drop little words of advice about fat or red meat. One quote I remembered was, "If it tastes good, spit it out." Lat was notorious for his diet and exercise routine; he was extremely disciplined about both. I was overcome with guilt. I made up my mind that night to do whatever I could to help even one person avoid my foolish mistakes. If I could get just one person to make lifestyle changes before it was too late, then all of my pain and suffering would have been worth it. I knew I needed to write to Lat when I got home.

Don't ignore the people that God places right in front of you. They are there for a reason. For me, they are usually the ones I don't like, or they irritate me for no apparent reason. Be careful, observe, and figure out what you are supposed to learn from them. It just might keep you off the transplant list.

On top of all the testing to get on the transplant list, there are many other issues to consider. There are financial issues, the surgery itself, post-operative care, rejection and immune system issues, and post-transplant lifestyle changes. It takes days to comprehend everything involved with a transplant. By the time I went through all of this, I wasn't really convinced this was such a great option. "God," I prayed, "some supernatural healing would be welcome now."

My case first had to be submitted to the Sanger Clinic's transplant committee for approval. I was told that not all cases passed this first hurdle. A heart transplant is considered the last resort. If the committee believes there are any other suitable options, the case will not be approved. Part of me believed I would not get over this first hurdle. Upon Sanger Clinic's approval, the case was then submitted to the insurance company for approval. After all, somebody had to come up with the $700,000, give or take a few thousand, to pay for this new heart. Assuming the insurance company approves this *minor* expenditure, your case goes to UNOS (United Network for Organ Sharing). UNOS is a non-profit organization that manages the organ transplant system, under contract with the federal government. It took about two months from start to finish to get listed with UNOS.

I was discharged a couple of days later with a list of exams, doctors, dentists, and optometrists to track down for the transplant committee. It felt like every day for two weeks I went to a different doctor to get something. I gave my taxi drivers a workout collecting all this information.

My dentist turned out to be the only hiccup, as he wanted to do a deep-tissue cleaning before signing off. He felt like some of my molars might be susceptible to abscess once my immune system was suppressed. It would be a two-step process, with half of my mouth worked on each visit. The nurse asked if next Thursday would be good for the first cleaning. Without thinking,

I agreed, not realizing that day was my birthday. I, Lord of the Idiots, made a dental appointment on my birthday.

The next Thursday rolled around, and I got a ride to the dentist's office. I got out of the car, took two steps, and felt very light-headed. I thought, "I'm going to faint really soon if I don't sit down." As I got closer to the door, reality started to slip away. I opened the door, sat down on the first chair, and immediately passed out (one might say died). Thank God nobody was in the waiting room. Two shocks later, which I thankfully didn't feel, I awoke to the TV showing Fox News. I immediately thought, "That's not what I was watching," as I had remembered being at a baseball field watching kids play and getting into an argument over whether or not I was supposed to be there. Coming back to reality is always such a pleasant experience. It's nice to know you didn't die again, and your heart is beating much more smoothly.

I waited about 15 minutes to make sure everything was OK before I checked in. After 15 more minutes they called me back, and I slowly walked to the chair.

I explained to the assistant that I had an episode out in their waiting room, and she might want to keep an extra eye on me today. She took my blood pressure, which was normal, gave me oxygen, and leaned me back in the chair. As the dentist numbed my mouth, the shots started to look a lot more intimidating than they actually were. I asked her to give me some nitrous gas to settle my anxiety.

Halfway through the procedure, the dentist stopped for a break. I looked at the assistant and told her that I was feeling a little nauseated, so she sat me up in the chair. Then I looked at her and said, "Now I'm feeling really nauseated." She handed me a wastebasket and turned off the nitrous. As soon as I saw that wastebasket, breakfast came up about eight times. I think everything made it into the wastebasket and very little clean up was needed in aisle 8. After a few minutes of pure oxygen, I felt better. The dentist came back in and finished without any more excitement.

I came home, sat down to relax, and thought, "I'm the only idiot on the planet that makes a dental appointment on his birthday, dies in the waiting room, and then pukes in the dentist chair." Note to self: No more dentist appointments on my birthday.

On Wednesday, September 9, I was heading back from a breakfast meeting. I looked over to Scott, my designated driver, and said, "Scott, I think I'm having an arrhythmia," because by now I was pretty good at sensing these things. As soon as I said it, I felt my ICD deliver a shock. Scott looked at me, I looked at him, and we both wondered what to do. I told him to just get me home. I'd call the doctor's office, as I already had a 3:00 appointment that day.

When I got to the doctor's office, they "interrogated" my ICD, which meant they downloaded the information from it. The guy from Biotronik shook his head while reading the printout. I said, "Mitch, what's up?" He looked at me and said, "Since August 18, the last time we interrogated your device, you've had 24 episodes." I looked at him and asked, "Is that a lot?" He just rolled his eyes and went to find the doctor.

Dr. Mehta came in and also shook his head. He said, "Do you know that you've had 24 episodes since August 18, and you have been shocked three times?" I told him that I'd heard, and I asked whether that was a lot. He rolled his eyes and said, "The next time you get shocked, call us. We are going to do an ablation on you. We need to get these arrhythmias under control." I thought to myself, "There's the understatement of the year." Always the smart aleck, but if we can't have fun going through this kind of thing, why go through it at all?

The next day, September 10, I had a neurological exam to make sure they were going to put a new heart into a body that had some brain control and could pass a field sobriety check. On the way there, I looked at my designated driver, Stephen, and said, "I think I'm having an arrhythmia." I waited for the shock, but it never came. The ICD "paced" me out of the episode. I called the doctor's office, believing that it hadn't shocked me yet, but it was probably just a matter of time. We might as well schedule the ablation and get it over with. After a few phone calls, they told me to come to the hospital. ,A room would be waiting for me.

So I went into the hospital to be observed, scare nurses, and wait for Dr. Mehta's schedule to clear up, which was a week later. Prior to my operation, I asked the nurse, "Is there any way this operation could make my arrhythmias worse?" She looked at me and said, "Art, you are already worse. Trust me, you are on the radar screen at the Sanger Clinic." Around 10:30 that morning, they took me to the pre-operative area. Everyone there was either waiting to get in the operating room or had just come out of the operating room. It was also chillier down there, and they really didn't like to hear the phrases, "I saw the light," or, "Just follow the light." Of course, I had to say them both, only to be reprimanded. Those people needed a little sense of humor down there.

Around noon, it was my turn to go to the operating room. As they wheeled me out of the holding pattern, a nice African-American female minister asked me if I would like some prayer. I wondered if she really had to ask at this point; I figured she could see the fear of God all over my face. I grabbed her hand and said, "Ma'am, give it your best shot!" She prayed, I prayed, and then I was off to the operating room.

The operating room was even colder than the pre-operative room. Upon my entrance, two attractive females introduced themselves and told me they were part of the anesthesiology team. I thought, "God, that sure was a fast answer! I must have died even before the operation began!" One lady leaned down and asked me if I had my "dream" picked out yet. If only I didn't have this gown on! Of course, I told her yes, my dream was a brown-eyed girl on the beach. How hard can it be to deliver this dream? About that time she put a mask over my face, and out went the lights.

About seven hours later, I woke up to a vision of the racquetball court at the YMCA. I was there with Billy Evans and his son Jay. Where was the beach? Where was the brown-eyed girl? I was so disappointed that the anesthesiology team had not delivered the dream I had ordered. By the time I got back to the recovery room, I was shaking off the effects of the anesthesia. I realized it felt like my groin had been hit by a hand grenade. A little bit later, Dr. Mehta came in to explain the seven hours of ablation surgery in terms he thought a seventh-grader could understand. He put a catheter up both sides of my groin, steered it into my heart, and started ablating (cauterizing) electrical areas that were causing arrhythmias. Naturally, to find those areas they have to put your heart into an arrhythmia. He said they only had to do this about seven times, so they only had to shock me out of the arrhythmias seven times. I thought, "That's why the brown-eyed girl never showed up. Who likes a lightning storm?"

During this time, my friends and family were getting very concerned about these life-and-death arrhythmias. Honestly, so was I. Some people thought it must be something I was doing, and I should stop doing whatever was causing them. Some people understood that my ICD had to be fine-tuned. I tried to explain to people if the doctors knew what caused the arrhythmias, they would tell me to stop doing it. Trust me, nobody wanted them to stop more than I did. No matter what I did or did not do, I had them. I could be riding in a car, walking the dog, or just eating a meal. It was one of the most frustrating experiences of my life. I realized everyone had the same goal; it was just a matter of how we got there.

I went home after the operation and had four days without arrhythmias. I was starting to think they had eliminated the problem, but the arrhythmias came back on the fifth day with a vengeance. On September 23, I entered a VT storm and had 49 episodes over three days. I felt every one of them. My ICD had recorded 91 events since it was implanted at the end of June. I was thinking I deserved a statue at the Biotronik headquarters, or at least a plaque. As a result, a second ablation surgery was scheduled.

As I sat in the waiting room hoping to get checked into a room quickly, I realized this would be my fourth hospital stay in the past four months. I told my sister Pat in Ohio that I was going back into the hospital, and I broke down on the phone. I was not looking forward to another week of needle sticks, poking, prodding, and being woken up at all hours of the night. I was also very concerned what would happen if this ablation did not work. Even though I had maintained a pretty good attitude through most of this ordeal, the severity of my condition hit home all at once. The surgery ended up taking about 12 hours. In recovery, my friend Billy asked me if I needed anything. I had not anything to eat or drink in 30 hours, and I was starving. The first thing that popped out of my mouth was, "Pizza!" Somebody went and got me two slices of pizza from Sbarro's. I had just bitten into my first slice of real food when in walked Dr. Mehta. If looks could kill, I think he would have been arrested for murder. The guy had just spent 12 hours inside my heart, and I'm munching on what turned out to be my last bite of pizza. I felt as guilty as he felt disappointed.

He said there would be no more ablation surgeries. He told me that when some people have an arrhythmia, their blood pressure drops slowly. In my case, however, every time they initiated an arrhythmia, my blood pressure dropped to zero immediately. I was glad he confirmed exactly what I had been experiencing. The next day, they wheeled in a TV with a DVD player. I proceeded to watch a movie on all the great aspects of an LVAD: a left ventricle assist device. This is a pump for your heart, and it needs to be inserted via open-heart surgery. It is battery-powered with two wires coming out of your side, and these batteries have to be changed every few hours. I thought, "Energizer bunny, here I come!" If this ablation surgery didn't work, this was where I was headed.

After a couple of days of recovery, I was discharged. I was a free man - sort of. That was October 1, 2009. They scheduled a six-week follow-up visit for November 9. I got to my check-up, thinking the last six weeks had been great with no shocks, no episodes, no runs, and no errors. I knew, however, that there had been some irregular heartbeats and palpitations. I thought there was a slight chance I'd get my driving privileges back, and I would truly be a free man. But Dr. Gulati thought it would be a good idea to get my device interrogated and see what the activity looked like.

About an hour later, Todd from Biotronik came in and did his thing. I felt proud because I knew nothing was going to show up, so I asked, "Todd, how is it looking?" He said, "Art, you've had 91 episodes in the last 41 days." I said, "Get out of here! You've got the wrong device - I've been fine."

He gave me the breakdown: 67 of the episodes had been in the range of 100-150 beats per minute, which required no therapy by the device. Of those, 14 were VTs and 10 were SVTs, all of which were paced out. Then he said, "You are up to 184 episodes since the end of June." I was thinking I should have that Biotronik plaque any day now. Is somebody calling Guinness with this? Since my driving privileges were headed out the door, I wondered how they might feel about me riding my motorcycle. Fortunately, these arrhythmias were not as serious as the ones I experienced prior to surgery; they did not warrant shocking my heart.

So the official answer was that I couldn't drive for six months after the last time my ICD shocked me. If all went well, March seemed like a good time to get behind the wheel. Until then, it was more time with Oprah and Dr. Phil. I couldn't wait to increase my wealth of useless information.

Chapter Eight

HEALING

With multiple cardiac emergencies over the last 16 years, I've spent a lot of time in hospital rooms, labs, doctors' offices, and emergency rooms. This has given me time to reflect on what is good for you, as well as what is not so good for you.

<u>First, healing is best done at home</u>. I think it is nearly impossible to heal in a hospital. Hospitals are great for some things, like emergency room care, delivering babies, and surgeries. After all the exciting stuff is done, however, to actually heal, regain strength, and let your body recover, I think you really need to be home.

There are numerous reasons for this. First, a hospital is a building full of sick people. How many germs are housed in this facility? If I were a germ, hanging out at the hospital would be like staying at the Biltmore. I would really like to know how all of the doctors, nurses, and other workers remain healthy in this environment.

Second, hospital food Stinks. Who could actually survive, let alone heal, eating hospital cuisine? Hello, nutrition, anybody home? Where does this stuff come from? Have you ever seen the "hospital diet" on Oprah? Nobody with any common sense would ever try it. Have you ever seen a doctor eating from a meal tray? No, they know better. All the nurses and visitors know the food in the cafeteria is much better than what they serve the patients. You would think for $1,500 a day I could get room service from the Grove Park Inn. Would somebody please inform the medical community of the nutrition/healthy body connection! Is it asking too much for just a few servings a day of fresh fruits and vegetables, as opposed to mass-produced instant mashed potatoes, cereal with no milk, processed hamburger steaks, and some sugar-laden dessert? Some of us don't want to be pill-popping robots for the rest of our lives.

Third, a positive attitude is paramount. This may be more important than anything I've written about so far. I was fortunate in my early business career to work for one of the most positive thinkers in the world. It didn't *all* rub off on me, as I naturally questioned, doubted, and had a healthy skepticism, but in the end I determined that attitude was a decision. I could be positive, or I could be negative. I figured I'd get out of the hospital sooner if I decided to be positive rather than negative.

I know I could have very easily justified adopting a victim mentality through all this. I could have given up somewhere along the line, and nobody would have blamed me. I mean, look at my resume; it's hardly the picture of success.

- Orphan at 17.
- Heart disease at 37.
- Divorced at 42.
- Fired at 42.
- Open-heart surgery at 42.
- Started a business and failed for two years.
- Obese at 47.
- Died at 51.

Who in their right mind would sign up for that? Here is another way to look at all of this.

- I survived the deaths of my parents.
- I graduated from college and earned a CPA certificate.
- I was married for 18 years and was blessed with three wonderful kids.
- I lost 65 pounds in a year and kept it off.
- I was blessed with surviving my own death.

Life is going to throw numerous things your way, across the spectrum from death, disease, depression, break-ups, disappointment, etc., all the way to love, joy, peace, contentment, happiness, etc. The key to success is how you respond to all of these situations.

In the hospital, I made up my mind that I was going to enjoy this adventure as much as I possibly could. I really considered it just another chapter in this journey called life. I wanted the doctors and nurses to realize I was different than most of their other patients. I wanted to bless the medical workers as much as all my family and friends blessed me. I knew the doctors were going to make the best decisions they could, so the best thing for me to do was to accept it and get on with the job of healing. Whether it was drawing blood daily, scheduling heart catheterizations, slicing my jugular vein, or performing a 12-hour surgery, my attitude was "Have at it."

One of my proudest moments in the hospital was when my cardiologist said he wanted to do this, this, and this. I looked at him and said, "Sure. Let's do it." He looked at me and said, "Art, you are not like any of my other patients." I asked, "What do you mean?" He replied, "When I tell my other patients I want to do some procedure, they get scared and worry. They think it's a matter of life and death. You are always willing, and you accept what I want to do." It made me feel good that he noticed my attitude.

In addition to having a positive mental attitude (PMA) and acceptance, I realized that a little gratitude goes a long way. This point was driven home when I finally got to talk to Dr. Ramos at the E.R., and I thanked him for saving my life. He was the one who said I was only the fourth person in 20 years to thank him. Not only was I only the fourth to thank him, but he could recall the first three immediately. Can you imagine working anywhere for 20 years, pouring your heart into your work, spending years to get educated, and you only get thanked four times in 20 years? This is a guy saving lives, mending broken bones, stitching up cuts, etc., and all he hears is people complaining and cussing him out. It doesn't take much gratitude to stand out in America today.

Being grateful stood out even more when I finally tracked down the two EMTs who saved my life at the Y. I always wondered about the guys that worked on me that night. A year passed before I finally decided to visit the hospital to request a copy of my medical records. I had never done this before, but how hard could this be? I knew the file would be quite thick, and I had no clue which records I might need to have copied. I made my request, which meant filling out several pages of paperwork. Somebody obviously saw the size of my file and came to my rescue. This wonderful person asked what I was doing and I told her I needed some backup for a book I was writing. She advised me that I only needed the doctor's notes and the ER report. Perfect! Two weeks and $100 later, I had my medical records. Lo and behold, there in the ER report, was the EMT report with names and a timeline.

Lauren, my daughter, was the one with the great idea. "Facebook them, Dad," she suggested, and so I did. I found Ricky Benson on Facebook and sent a friend request. I was hoping he was the right Ricky Benson. He was elated to hear from me, and I scheduled a lunch with him and his partner, Matt Hoyle.

During lunch, both of them said that they never hear from any of their "saves." Ricky said he had been an EMT for 31 years, and I was the first person to ever thank him. Matt had been an EMT for nine years, and he said this lunch would keep him going for another 10 years. I didn't know what to say to these people who saved my life, other than, "Thank you." It seems so meaningless, but it meant everything in the world to these two guys. When I told them I was writing a book and asked them about to write a foreword, they responded enthusiastically: Yes! These people are unsung heroes. They spend their lives saving others, get paid very little, and receive minimal amounts of recognition or thanks. Why are the most valuable people in our society sometimes the most under paid and least appreciated?

Be thankful for everything – the good and the bad. In 1 Thessalonians 5:18, the Bible says, *"Give thanks in all circumstances, for this is God's will for you in Christ Jesus."* Notice it says *all* things, not just the good things. Ephesians 5:20 says the same thing, *"Always giving thanks to God the Father for everything, in the name of our Lord Jesus Christ."* Again, it says everything, not just some things. Is everything really everything? Yes! When they tell you that you need a new heart, thank Him. When they draw blood at 3:00 a.m., thank Him. When they stitch you up, thank Him. When they rescue you at the YMCA, thank Him. When your car gets wrecked, thank Him. When you lose a job, thank Him. When you want to lash out at the world because life isn't fair, thank Him. God knows what He is doing, although it might be years before you know why something "happened" in your life.

Thank the people around you. So few people ever get thanked for the jobs they do. Be on that doctor's list of patients who ever gave thanks. Be the first on that EMT's list of "saves" who ever gave thanks.

Be different. Do you realize that if you are just appreciative and thankful most of the time, you will be different from most people? I wanted to be different in the hospital. I chose to be as happy and as upbeat as I could, given the circumstances. I made a conscious decision, no matter whether I lived or died in the hospital. I wanted the nurses, doctors, and assistants to know that I was different. I knew that I was surrounded with sick, dying, or unhealthy patients and families that were upset. I knew the same thing surrounded the people that worked there every day. For me, being happy and thankful was not that big of a challenge. I knew that if God could pull me through cardiac arrest, He could get me through the rest of my hospital visits. He can do the same for you!

Be grateful to those who spend long hours helping others. Count your blessings, not your sorrows.

Most people expect doctors and nurses to be perfect. It's almost as if we have conferred "God" status upon the medical world and believe they are miracle workers. We set the bar so high that if they don't reach it, or, God forbid, make a mistake, it's time to call the attorneys. Remember, they are human. They are not perfect. They are not God, although I'm sure some doctors might disagree. They will make a mistake now and then. I just have to remember that I have made plenty of mistakes in my lifetime. I admire and respect their dedication and devotion to the profession. These people have spent years learning and educating themselves, so I respect and value their opinions accordingly. That does not mean, however, they have carte blanche over my life and body. As a matter of fact, I had one doctor tell me, "Art, you're the only patient I have that tells *me* what we are going to do." He then asked me where I got my medical degree. I told him, "The University of Sears. Where did you get yours?" I asked. Without batting an eye, he said, "The University of Wal-Mart." Sometimes you just have to laugh at life.

Fourth, healing takes faith and prayer. I did not have a lot of faith prior to June 11. I believed in God, Jesus, and the Holy Spirit, but they were handling the big issues of the day; I didn't feel like I was even on the radar screen. After all, who am I? Once I could comprehend the events of June 11 and His amazing grace towards me, I had no doubt that God had me firmly in His hand. That made all the events I had to face in the coming months so much easier. It also allowed me to have a good attitude about this whole thing (most of the time). I knew that no matter what I faced, it was in God's hands, so I might as well enjoy it.

That doesn't mean I was fearless, or that I didn't worry, about my situation. I had plenty of worries, and I think most people would, too. Every time a doctor came in with results, or wanted to try another procedure, or my heart didn't beat right (which it did quite often and still does), a little worry or fear would show up. I had to consciously remind myself who was in charge. If I could get through June 11 with His help, then this too would pass.

Life and death were staring me in the face every day I was in the hospital. Would I wake up tomorrow? Would I get shocked again? How much longer would I live? How long would my heart last? Could I survive another operation? It went on 24 hours a day. Without faith, I could have very easily succumbed to these thoughts. Faith is believing in the unseen. It doesn't take any faith to believe the things we see; that's easy. On the other hand, how hard is it to believe you will thrive, when all the reports and professionals say otherwise?

I think it took something catastrophic for Him to get my attention. It was just another reminder that my mission was not complete.

I had to come to grips with the fact that God was in control. It was a lot easier to accept that fact in the hospital, when I was clueless about what was going to happen from moment to moment. As soon as I started worrying about something, I reminded myself that God, not Art, is in control. For a bean counter like me, that is a lot easier said than done. It's not easy changing 50-year-old behaviors and thoughts. However, I was in the perfect place to learn that lesson.

Without faith in something bigger than yourself,

you'll probably be on a rollercoaster like I was. Once you accept the fact that you are not in control, and the temporary nature of this world, you can take everything that life throws you in stride. We are only in this world for a moment, compared to eternity. My dad used to take my mom past a church sign every time she got upset about something. It always read, "Count your blessings, not your sorrows." You can spend your time focused on all your problems and drama, or you can focus on the solution and look for the best in a situation. It's a choice, and you have the freedom to decide.

The things or situations we get upset about are usually meaningless. It's just "stuff" that you won't take with you when you die. The only things of lasting value on this earth are love and relationships. Put that problem or situation in its proper perspective. Compared to eternity, does it really matter? Wouldn't it be better for your soul to handle problems with honor and grace, as opposed to anger and outrage? Trust me, I've been angry and outraged. Just ask my family. It does not help your heart, nor does it help your soul.

Once I realized that nothing, not even death, could resist the will of God, it was a lot easier to accept situations that came my way. I knew for certain that God had my life firmly in His grasp. He has your life in His grasp as well. He is a big God, bigger than we think. So when your arrhythmias of life come, you hit your concrete curb face-first, or you need something transplanted in your life, remember whose hands you are in. I know the situation might be fearful, lonely, or discouraging. However, when you remind yourself who is in charge, you will have peace that surpasses all understanding.

I have spent most of my life worrying about things that, 97% of the time, never materialized. I worried about confrontations, and I tried to think of every conceivable argument or comeback. I worried about bills and how to pay them. Some of them never even showed up.

Being a trained CPA, I had every penny budgeted I thought would come my way for the next two years. Imagine my resentment when something showed up that was not in the budget. I spent a lifetime being frustrated over the unbudgeted items of my life. Just when I thought there would be some money to save at the end of the month, the car broke down, the washing machine needed to be fixed, or the roof leaked.

I had always lived my life in the future. Today was never enough. It didn't matter that I had a roof over my head, food in the refrigerator, and a car to drive. I took those luxuries for granted. The really important stuff was in the future, just waiting for me. Imagine my shock when I came across the following from Matthew 6: 25-34.

DO NOT WORRY

Therefore I tell you, do not worry about your life, what you will eat or drink; or about your body, what you will wear. Is not life more important than food, and the body more important than clothes? Look at the birds of the air; they do not sow or reap or store away in barns, and yet your heavenly Father feeds them. Are you not much more valuable than they? Who of you by worrying can add a single hour to his life?

And why do you worry about clothes? See how the lilies of the field grow. They do not labor or spin. Yet I tell you, not even Solomon in all his splendor was dressed liked one of these. If that is how God clothes the grass of the field, which is here today and tomorrow thrown into the fire, will He not much more clothe you? O you of little faith? So do not worry, saying, 'What shall we eat?' or 'What shall we drink?' or 'What shall we wear?' For the pagans run after all these things and your heavenly Father knows you need them. But seek first his kingdom and his righteousness, and all these things will be given to you as well. Therefore do not worry about tomorrow, for tomorrow will worry about itself. Each day has enough trouble of its own.

Now, when all the worries of this life inevitably come, I implement the 24-hour rule. If I am worried about something for more than a day or a night, I have to read the above and let it go. As a matter of fact, if I had my way, I would make the above verses standard provisions on all birth certificates, marriage licenses, and home mortgages!

In addition to faith, there is prayer. I cannot tell you the thousands of people, whom I will never meet, who prayed for me. The number of people that I *did* know or know of who prayed for my recovery was even amazing. I am the perfect example of God answering prayers. He may not always answer them in our time frame or with the outcome we desire, but God does answer prayers. I also had numerous visitors that prayed with me before leaving, which was a great blessing. I had this picture in my mind of all these prayers for me going up and God saying, "OK, I've got the Townsend case handled! Can we please go on to something else? How about world hunger?" I was so thankful for everyone's persistence; it definitely helped the survival and healing process.

Fifth, music heals. The music on my iPhone was as critical to me as the heart monitors. I used my iPod at all times of the day or night. Music has the ability to touch your mind and soul, bringing out healing emotions and thoughts that nothing else can touch. Music calmed me down several times and helped me sleep every night. For the most part, I listened to contemporary Christian musicians, like Jesus Culture from California. The message of God, love, grace, mercy, and healing had a great impact on my body and soul. Music really should be part of your daily life; it's that important. I cannot imagine getting out of the hospital sooner without it.

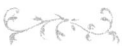

A wonderful friend once told me, "Miracles happen quickly, and healing takes a little longer." My desire is for nobody to have to spend any significant time in a hospital. Hospitals can be a scary place, especially when the outcome is unknown. Wouldn't it be wonderful if we were so healthy that hospitals were no longer needed? If you do find yourself or a loved one there, I hope you will find some comfort in the words above.

Chapter Nine
TIME'S UP

Train a child in the way he should go and when he is old he will not turn from it.
Proverbs 22:6

That statement is true, but it doesn't address the time between being a child and being old. For me, the in-between time was the difference between night and day. Having gone to church every Sunday for 17 years, I felt pretty qualified for the training part. I learned a lot about the Bible. I knew most of the stories in the Old and New Testament. I knew about Moses, Noah, David, Samson, and Solomon. I knew about Jesus, his miracles and parables, his death, and his resurrection. I knew he was the Son of God and that he died for everyone's sins. I believed it was all true - true for everybody but me.

If God really loved me, why was I an orphan at 17? If God really loved me, why was I in so much pain after the deaths of my parents? If God really loved me, why did all my relationships end in pain, usually my own? If God really loved me, why did He always take away the people I loved? If God really loved me, why didn't I feel it? It went on and on.

I had some knowledge of God because my parents were diligent about church attendance. But I didn't *know* God. I knew information about God, but I didn't have a relationship with Him. I had never had an encounter with Him, until June 11, 2009. Somewhere between the end of the first week and the start of the second week in the hospital, my short-term memory started coming back to me. Each day I could remember another piece of the "puzzle," and sometime after the first week I started to comprehend the miracles that had happened to me.

There was a light bulb moment. I could finally remember the stories of what had happened to me since I went into cardiac arrest at the Y. I immediately became overwhelmed with the grace and mercy of God, and I wept. I just couldn't believe God would do that for me. To me, grace is undeserved mercy. Nobody was more undeserving than me. There was not much I could point to in my life that warranted that kind of grace. "Me, of all people," I thought.

Not only was I the recipient of this extraordinary grace, but I hadn't even asked for it! I was dead. I couldn't talk, pray, or beg God to save my life. I had no thoughts I had no awareness of where I was or the situation I was facing. I did, however, have a lot of people praying for me, speaking life into the situation and asking God for his mercy. I'll never know all the people who prayed for me, but they obviously had a direct connection to God. Not only did God show up and spare my life, but He made sure I had no long-term brain damage and the blood clots in my brain dissolved naturally.

People always ask me what I "saw" or experienced when I was dead. I think they want to know what it's like to spiritually encounter God and Jesus Christ in the afterlife. I would love to write about that experience, but I have no memory of any such events. Based upon my first heart attack and experience, and my belief in the Bible, I do know that there is life after death.

Prior to June 11, 2009, I was admittedly skeptical whenever I heard someone say that God spoke to him or her. I had always thought that God was so Awesome, so Holy, and so Supreme, who am I to receive any word from God? Growing up, I knew that if God was going to speak to me, it had to be through a burning bush, a choir of angels, or a voice so loud everyone would hear it.

I eventually got control of my emotions and asked God over and over, "Why me?" I must have asked this for hours that day. Finally, I think God got tired of hearing my questions and answered me directly with, "Time's up." I would like to say this was a big, booming voice from Heaven, and everyone in the room heard it, but it wasn't. I wish I could speak about a vision of Heaven and all the glory, but that would not be true, either. What I heard and felt was simply on the inside of me. He said, "Art, your time was up, and I saved you. There are things in your life that I have told you to end, and you had not done them. Time's up." I knew immediately what He was talking about. Then He continued, "Time's up for everybody. People who have one foot in church and one foot in the world need to make a decision. Parents who have not spoken to their children, who keep putting off difficult conversations until next week: time's up. Spouses who haven't spoken truthfully to each other: time's up. You don't have tomorrow; all you have is right now. I am coming back and will separate the wheat from the chaff. Time's up."

Nobody knows when He is coming back, and I certainly do not profess to know. The words He spoke to me were one thing; the overwhelming sense of urgency that was impressed upon me was so much more real. I had never felt a greater sense of urgency in my life. I knew immediately at least one thing I needed to finish. It probably doesn't sound like a big deal, but I felt like God wanted me to end a particular business relationship in the months prior to June 11. I was moving in that direction, but not as fast as I should have been. This relationship had been very profitable over the past 10 years, so ending it wasn't easy. Looking back now, God obviously wanted to speed up the process.

Nothing can resist the will of God. It doesn't matter what life-and-death situation you are facing, whether it's a car wreck, a heart attack, a gunshot or a disease;

if it's not God's will, then you are staying right here in this world. Your mission is not complete.

I love the message of, "Time's up." It can be applied to almost every area of your life. It's about not putting off until tomorrow, next week, or next month what you should do or say because you may never see that day. It's about dealing with life right now. Nobody has promised us tomorrow, but most of us spend our lives worrying and planning for some future event and ignore the present.

How different would we treat each other if we consciously focused on the thought, "Time's up?" What if this is the last time you pass this way? If you knew for certain this was the last time you'd ever see your son, daughter, or spouse, how would you treat them? What would you want to say to them? Time's up! If it were the last time to see your husband, would you really be upset that he left the toilet seat up? If it were the last time to see your wife, would you really be upset that she bought a coat that was on sale? If it were the last time to see your son, would you be upset he didn't mow the grass yet? If it were the last time to see your daughter, would you be upset that she came in late last night? If it were the last day on the job, would you be complaining about the copier or your co-worker? If it were the last time to see your father, would you be upset he took your cell phone away?

If we knew for certain something was going to be the last time ever, wouldn't we act a bit differently?

What are the unsaid truths you would want them to know? Time's up! Say it now. You might not have next week to tell your spouse how much you love them. Whatever you're afraid to say, say it now. Time's up! Whatever you don't want to confront, confront it now. Time's up! Whatever you don't want to do, do it now. Time's up! Whatever decision you're putting off, decide it now. Time's up!

I know that life's tragedies happen when it's "just another day." I cannot think of one tragedy in my life that I actually "planned." I never woke up and said, "Today is a great day for a heart attack," or, "Today is just a wonderful day for a car wreck," or, "Today is a good day to die." How many of us are living in the future, unconscious to what is happening right now? You don't have to die to wake up, unless you have to be beat over the head with multiple near-death experiences like me. I don't mean that you need to adopt a morbidity mentality and become clinically depressed. I'm just saying how much better off we, and the world, would be if we adopted an attitude of more love, kindness, and truthfulness? What if we showed a little more gratitude towards others and realized, "Time's up?" Maybe we would act a little better, have a little more patience, show a little more love, and have just a tiny bit more compassion for others? So many of us, including myself, just assume our wives or husbands will walk in the door at night, our kids will always be safe, our jobs will always be there, and our parents will live forever.

I'm not suggesting this has to be in our thoughts 24 hours a day. However, the next time you start to complain or get angry, stop and put things in perspective. There are no guarantees in life, and you might only be passing this way once.

Chapter Ten

WHATEVER LIFE I HAVE LEFT, I WANT TO SPEND IT LIVING

Prior to my ablation surgeries in September of 2009, I was literally living moment-to-moment. I never knew when another arrhythmia would happen. I could not commit to do anything without the caveat of, "If I am having a good day." Every time I felt my heart miss a beat or get out of rhythm, which I could now discern immediately, I immediately wondered if this was my time to go. I fearfully anticipated my ICD charging up and kicking me in the chest. Sometimes I looked around for a soft place to land, so I wouldn't hit a concrete curb. When I was discharged for the last time at the end of September, I had no idea what to expect.

I prayed my arrhythmias would cease and the last ablation surgery would be a success, however that was defined. Dr. Mehta told me there were no guarantees. He said some lasted a week, a month, or a year. He said the heart constantly looked for new electrical pathways, so there was no way to tell how long-lasting or successful the surgery would be. If this didn't stop the arrhythmias, the only option left, outside of a transplant, was to put an LVAD in my heart.

I despised the thought of getting an LVAD, as it meant another open-heart surgery. It also meant my life would be in the hands of charged-up batteries, and it would definitely lead to a heart transplant. This assumed a heart could be found, and it also meant yet another open-heart surgery. I had had such a horrible experience with my first open-heart surgery that one or two more surgeries within the same year seemed deplorable.

They reset my driving privileges after my last surgery for another six months, which meant my freedom would be restored at the end of March of 2010. During that period, I was blessed with many friends who took me to appointments, daily errands, and entertainment outings. I eventually had a list of people I could call. I was amazed at the generosity and giving nature of friends and family. If you want to find out who your friends are, just lose your driving privileges for about a year.

One of my regular drivers was Pastor Kathy from the Shield of Faith Church, Pastor Larry's wife. We were out on an errand one day, and she said one of her recommendations to people in my condition was to make a goal to travel. She said I should pick a place I had always wanted to see, and I should just go. At the time, I thought, "Just driving to the grocery store by myself would be a great goal." Even so, she had planted a seed, which was probably her intention all along. Over the next several weeks, I pondered her suggestion and knew the place I had always wanted to see was the "big hole," also known as the Grand Canyon.

As the days passed and I didn't get shocked or pass out, my confidence began to grow. I began to think that maybe my arrhythmias were gone for good. I could accept a lunch invitation for the following week and feel pretty confident that I would actually show up.

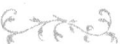

Setting Small Tasks/Goals

My son Matt became a frequent weekend visitor. In December, I noticed the headlight was out on his truck. I figured this was something so small that even I could fix it. I hitched a ride to the auto parts store and came home with a light bulb. It was cold and wet outside, but I thought I could handle about 15 minutes of it before my heart started acting up. In my mind, this would probably take five minutes at most.

I opened the hood and took the bad bulb out from in front of the battery. As soon as I got it out, I knew getting the new bulb in was going to be very challenging, due to the limited space. I spent almost 30 minutes outside trying unsuccessfully to get that bulb in place and hooked up to the wiring harness. I was cold and tired, and my heart was starting to act up. I was short of breath and could feel the palpitations. Prior to my ablation surgeries, this feeling would have accelerated into a full-blown arrhythmia. During an arrhythmia, my chest would feel hollow, then I'd get lightheaded and pass out as my blood pressure dropped to zero. That would all happen in a matter of two or three seconds. Defeated, I went back in the house.

I slumped down on the couch, depressed that I had failed at a task for my son. After about an hour, I was rested up and ready for one more shot with the bulb. Before going out, I had a little prayer with God. I said, "God, you know I can't get this bulb in. I don't have the strength or the patience. I want to do this so Matt won't get a ticket for having his headlight out. If this is going to happen, You are going to have to do it because I can't."

I went outside. As soon as I lifted up the hood, it started raining. I thought, "Great, now I'm wet *and* cold. God, I'm going to give this one shot, and then I'm out of here." I grabbed the bulb, inserted it into the socket, and it fit perfectly. The wiring harness slipped on without a problem, and I was done in less than a minute. I went into the house, completely stunned and dumbfounded.

I couldn't believe God would actually help me put in a light bulb. I told God, "I understand You handle the big things, like bringing me back from death, but You also help me install a meaningless light bulb?" Ever so clearly, I heard Him say, "Art, I want to be involved in every aspect of your life, from changing a bulb to bringing you back to life and everything in between." God is great; we need to call on him more often.

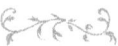

The Joy of Social Networks

I think one of the greatest things about social networking is getting in touch with long-lost people. In addition to this, it was a great way to keep everyone up-to-date on my condition. As a heart patient this saved me from having to share the same story over and over again. It also kept the prayer team informed. About this time, I was "Facebooked" by my long-lost "adopted" sister, Karen, from Mansfield, Ohio. I had not talked to her or her husband, Joe, in over 30 years. For several years after the deaths of my parents, I dated her younger sister. We had always assumed we would be brother and sister-in-law, but it was not to be. Regardless, Karen and Joe always treated me well and had opened their home to me numerous times when I was in the area. After I moved to Charlotte, we lost touch until the winter of 2009.

We were all thrilled to be re-connected on Facebook, and we exchanged numerous messages back and forth in an effort to update each other. They mentioned they would be heading to Florida in a couple of months. They wanted to stop by on the way home, and I naturally said yes.

I eagerly awaited their arrival two months later. I was curious how 30 years had treated them, and I'm sure they felt the same way about me. When they pulled into the driveway, I went outside to meet them. I hugged Karen, and to my astonishment, she looked like she was still in high school. I hugged Joe, and outside of a few extra pounds since his wrestling days, he looked great. We went into the living room and picked up right where we had left off 30 years ago. At dinner that night, Joe made a comment that really stuck with me. He said, "People always say one day they are going to do something. If you want to do something, do it now! Why wait for 'one day,' which may not ever happen?"

After they left, I kept thinking about Joe's comment and my plans to head out to the "big hole." It always amazes me how one seemingly innocent comment can change your life or point it in a different direction.

If we would just listen, those comments always seem to arrive right on time, usually from a source we least expect. I weighed the pros and cons of traveling 3,000 miles west and considered what the worst thing was that could happen. I also knew I had an unknown window of opportunity with my health. I came to the conclusion that whatever time I had left, I wanted to spend it living. I had spent almost a year without driving privileges and many weeks in and out of the hospital. Countless hours were spent wondering if every out-of-rhythm heartbeat was the last one. I also spent a lot of time thinking about if I would ever want or receive a new heart. I did not want to lie in a hospital bed, waiting for something to happen or not happen, and regret that I never saw the "big hole."

I could have easily given up. I could have stayed on my couch, collected disability checks, and waited to get worse. The only way to move up the transplant list was to get worse. I could have declared that I wasn't doing anything until I got a new heart. Instead, I made a conscious decision that I would focus on living, and not dying.

I looked at all areas of my life, from my relationship with God, my nutritional habits, my relationships (family, personal and professional), to even writing a book. I knew I could do a lot better in most of those areas. My mission became to give back. My goal was to prevent just one person from going through what I had gone

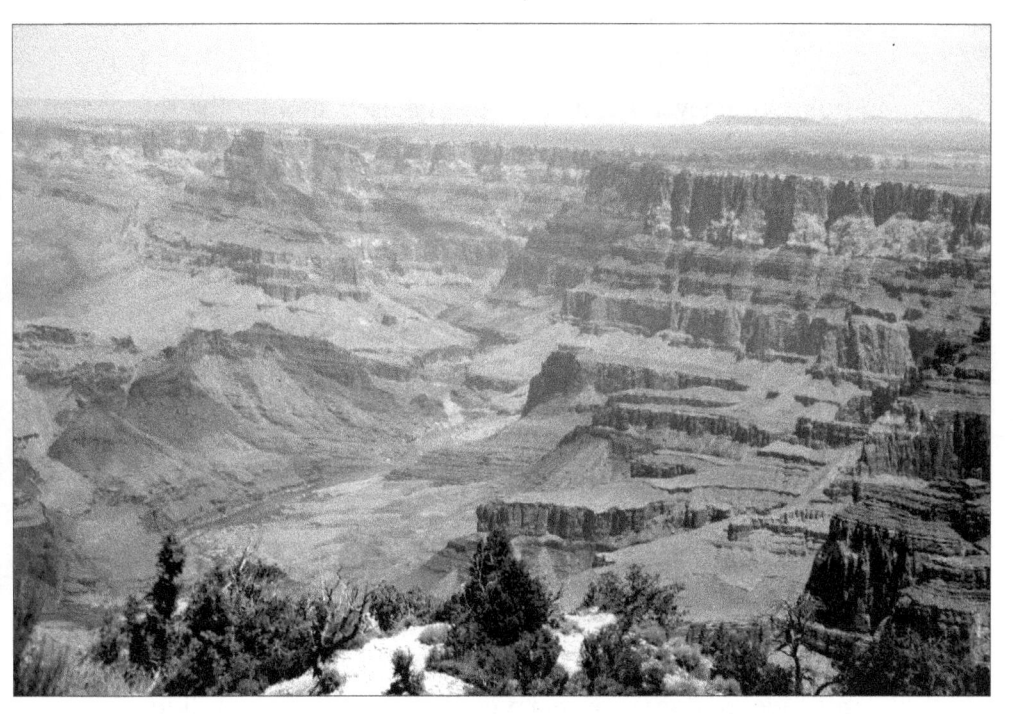

The Big Hole

through. Surely, somebody could avoid the mistakes I made. If I could change just one life, it would make all the pain worth it. I got involved in local charitable events, I helped out with a career transitions group, and I attended a men's ministry meeting every week. I spoke whenever I got invited. I raised money for the American Heart Association and won a lifestyle change award. I told my story to anyone who would listen. By now, I'm sure those around me were tired of hearing it.

Everyone told me God must have big plans for me. The more I thought about it, the more I realized God has big plans for everybody. I was just blessed to receive the gift from God of a second (well maybe third or fourth) chance that I did not want to squander. When your life expectancy can be measured more easily in months than years, it is amazing how your perspective on life changes. Suddenly, those daily concerns, like what I am going to wear, or when the house payment is due, aren't that important. Questions like, "Will I see my kids graduate or marry? Will I see my grandkids grow up? Will my spouse survive without me?" become much more paramount.

I have always said nobody lies on their deathbed and wishes they could have worked longer, closed one more deal, had one more client or performed one more surgery. What you do wish for is more time. Time to see your children grow. Time to say all those things that have been left unsaid over the years. Time to see all those things you promised yourself "some day" you would see. Time to live a life pleasing to God and be able to hear, "Well done, my good and faithful servant." Time to create that bucket list and actually check off some items. For me, that time was now. God had placed more sand in my hourglass, and I didn't want to waste a day feeling sorry for myself. I wanted to live, whether I had a week left or 30 years.

HEADING WEST

As I got closer to having my driving privileges restored, I became more vocal about heading to the Grand Canyon in June. The majority of people were very supportive, but there were a few folks who thought I had lost my mind. They were concerned about what we would do if something happened. Questions like, "What are you going to do if you need medical attention? What if the transplant team calls you with a new heart? Will the kids be able to fly out to Arizona if you are in a hospital?" I was concerned about all those issues and more. However, it always came down to, "If not now, when?" I knew anything could happen, but I felt like the probability was small. Each passing day without a shockable event increased my confidence. I prayed about the adventure as well. Every time I prayed about it, the only thing I heard was, "Go." I think God knew saying more than a few words might just confuse me. I wanted to make sure this wasn't just an "Art" thing, but the Big Guy was on board as well. I was learning that less of "Art" in something and more of God works out a lot better. "Art" had made enough mistakes on his own.

Another motivating factor for me to head west was the movie and book, *Into the Wild*. It is the true story of a young man, Christopher McCandless, and it depicts his two-year adventure of leaving society and living in the West and Alaska. I would recommend this book or movie for anybody who has a sense of adventure. In my heart, I yearned to head west on the road. I also decided "Into the Wild" would be the name of this latest adventure.

Somewhere along the line, someone mentioned that I should get an RV and haul my motorcycle with it. I had wanted an RV for years, but I could neither afford nor justify buying one. Still, the idea made me search online to see what was out there. I was shocked to see that prices had dropped nearly 30-40% in the recession. This changed my outlook on the trip; it went from just a motorcycle ride and motels to camping out across the country. Besides, if the world turned upside down, I'd always have a place to live.

It always amazes me that when I make a buying decision based on emotion, I try to justify it with logic. Combining emotions and logic into one decision is lethal. A few weeks later, there was an RV parked

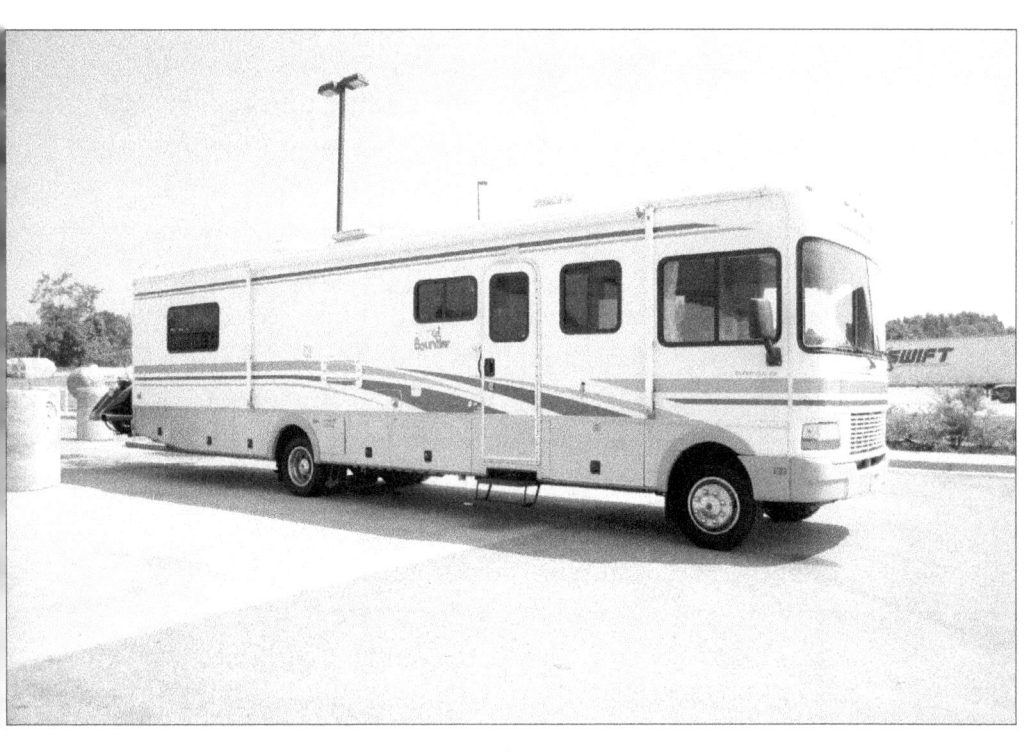

The Magic Bus

in the driveway, and my home equity line was nearly wiped out. A sane man, one who wasn't on the heart transplant list, would have probably been more rational than I was. There simply are times in your life when you have to follow your dreams, despite what the world might say. This seemed like one of those times.

Matt approached me about joining me on the trip. I readily agreed, and I was so excited to have him plan the trip with me. Of course, our planning only involved when we would leave and how long we would be gone. He quit his job and sold a dirt bike to have the funds to survive for a couple of months. We departed on June 24, 2010, almost a year to the day after I was released from the hospital after my cardiac arrest. We spent nearly two months on the road, traveled 9,500 miles, and saw most of the U.S.

The Grand Canyon was the physical highlight of the trip for me. I wish there were words that would do this marvel justice, but there aren't. I wish pictures could capture the breadth and depth of this majesty, but they don't. If you have never seen this wonderful creation of God, go! As a matter of fact, go now! Don't wait until the kids are older, or when you get around to it. Do not leave this Earth without seeing this wonder. If you ever need to feel the awesomeness of God, go to the Grand Canyon. Drive to the first overlook. Keep your head pointed down, and when you run into the railing at the end of the overlook, look up. Your mind will not comprehend what it sees. Your knees

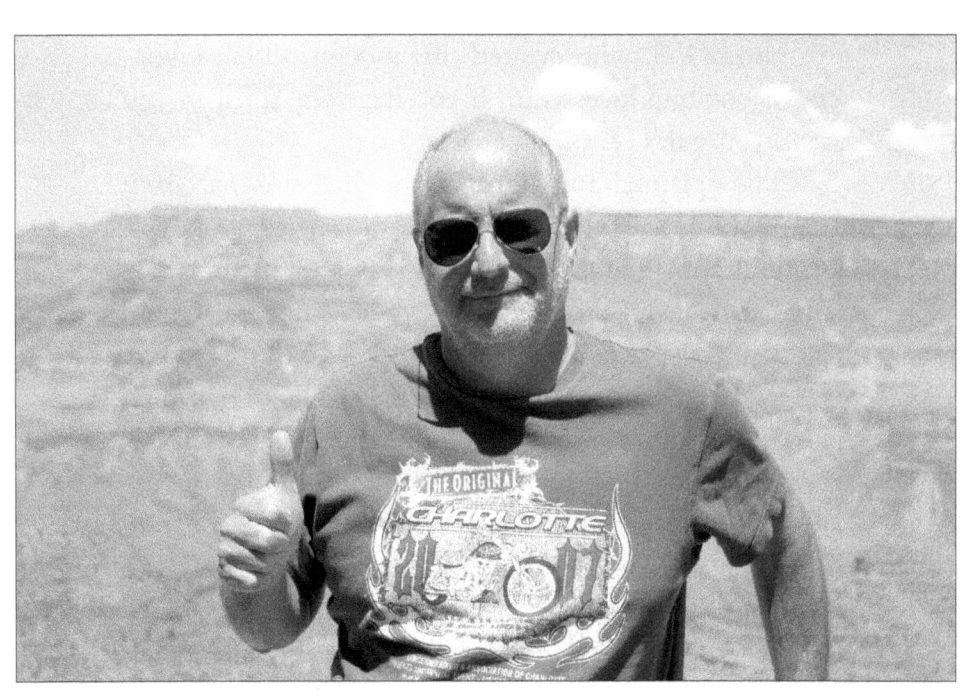

I finally made it to the Grand Canyon.

will buckle, and your eyes will fill up with tears. You will feel so insignificant and humble before the immenseness, which was created by the Creator of the entire universe. You will then be in awe and wonder that this same God, who created this indescribable canyon, knows you and loves you. If you have any spirit in you at all, you will cry. Well, at least I did.

The spiritual highlight of the trip was Salvation Mountain in Slab City, California. I learned about this location from *Into the Wild,* as it was one of the places Christopher McCandless discovered. After the Grand Canyon, this place was next on my list of things to see. It is located near the town of Niland, California, which is in the southeastern part of the state. Slab City is an old Marine base the government shut down in the 1960s. They demolished everything but the concrete slabs, hence the name. Over the years, it has been the year-round home of hippies, and in the winter snowbirds arrive from Canada. It is in the desert, and I warn you not to visit in July, like Matt and I did. When we were there, the temperature was 110 all day long, and at night it cooled off to 102.

Every now and then, you cross paths with someone special. It might be for a minute or two, but if you are lucky it lasts longer. In the depths of your soul there is a connection. Your spirit leaps, and your heart feels the love of God. That's exactly what happened the instant I met Leonard Knight.

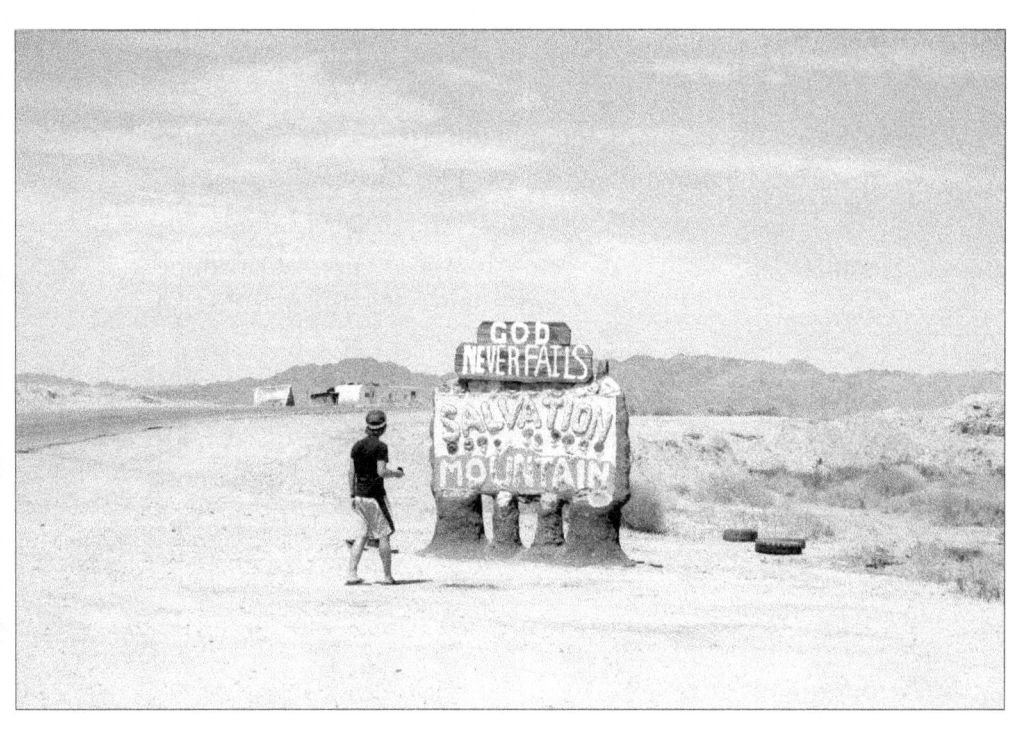

Matt at Salvation Mountain

As we approached the "God is love" mountain, we were greeted by a thin, older man with both of his arms raised to the sky, booming out, "Welcome! Come here. I'd like to show you something." We spent the next hour and a half with the creator of Salvation Mountain, Leonard Knight, on a personal tour of his creation. Leonard told us his life story and testimony. He has spent nearly 30 years in the desert building Salvation Mountain. He built the mountain out of adobe, concrete, and over 100,000 gallons of paint, all of which was donated. It stands about 100 feet tall, which doesn't sound like a lot. In the middle of the desert, this, and the fact that one man did it all, is very impressive. I'm not sure I've ever met a more gracious and humble host. Leonard has lived in Slab City all these years in the back of his pickup truck. At 78, Leonard's passion for God has not subsided one bit. He was so honored that we stopped to see Salvation Mountain, but we were the ones who were honored to be with him.

Leonard is a simple man with a simple message, "God is love." He has been trying to spread that message to the world for over 30 years. He has that childlike faith that the Gospel describes. There are no theology lessons or ulterior motives; there is just the simple thought that God is love. Leonard is one of those people you meet that reaffirms your faith in God. He exudes the love of God, and it is hard to be in his presence and not be touched. If you are ever in that area, it is well worth a trip to the desert to meet this man of God. Your heart and soul will thank you.

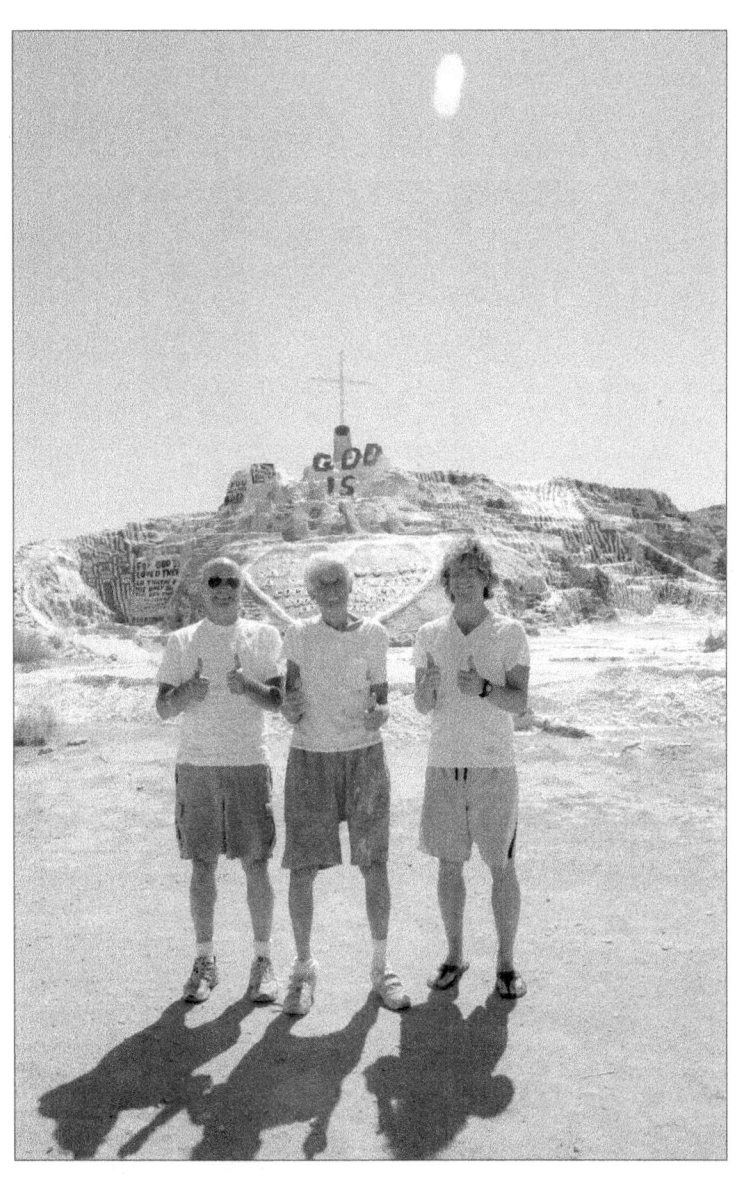

Matt and I with Leonard Knight (middle).

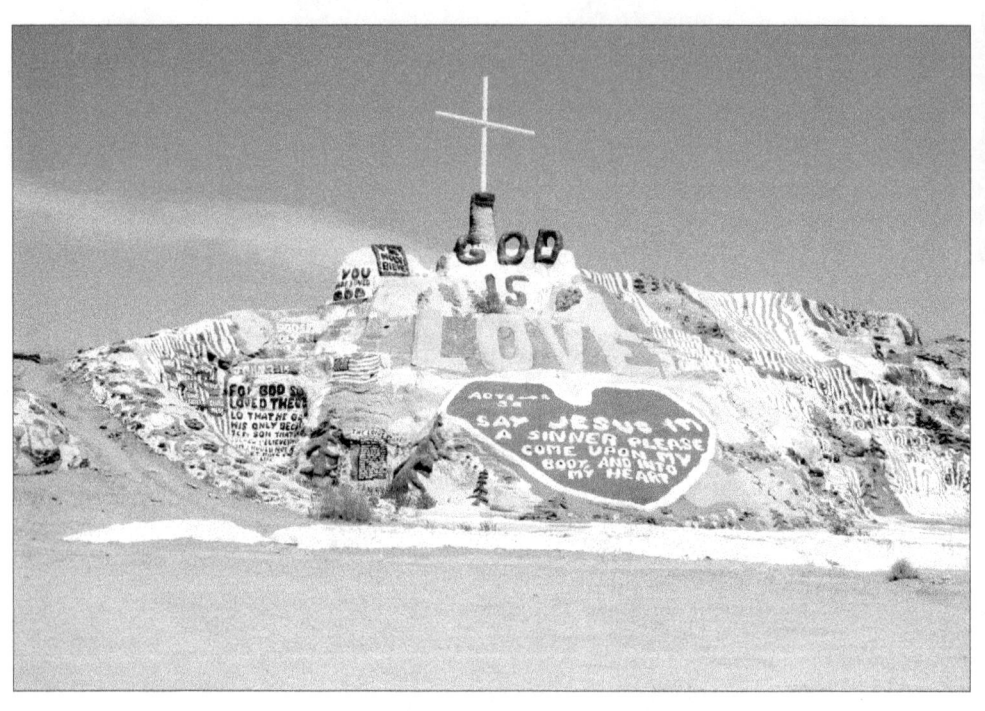

Salvation Mountain

I could have spent two more months exploring this wonderful country, but Matt needed to get home and find a job. We started this trip together; so we ended it together.

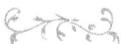

Eating Healthy

In addition to traveling, I focused a lot of my time and energy on eating healthfully and learning about our food supply. I found out the hard way that losing weight doesn't mean you are healthy. I watched the documentary, *Food, Inc.*, and it really changed how I look at food. It became quite clear to me that even eating the "right" foods, like fruits, vegetables, fish, white meat, beans, and nuts, could be harmful if they are filled with insecticides, pesticides, and growth hormones. I promise that if you watch *Food Inc.*, you will never go through another drive-thru or shop your local grocery store unless they have a great supply of organic goods. You will find a farmers market or local health food store instead. The sooner you understand the connection between food and health, the quicker you'll increase your longevity on this planet.

Think about it for a second. How many chemicals have you ingested over the years from the food you eat? Do you really want to eat something that has been genetically modified to withstand the application of Roundup weed killer? First, the vegetable or fruit had its DNA changed from how God created it. Second, it is covered with Roundup. Why put something like that in your body?

I have come to realize that I am responsible for my health. The medical community is not responsible for my health. There is not a pill made, nor will there ever be one made, that is going to cure bad eating habits, sedentary lifestyles, and a corrupt food supply. The government is not responsible for my health. The health insurance industry is not responsible for my health. Nobody ever held a gun to my head and forced me to eat barbeque, cheeseburgers, or pizza. What I choose to eat is literally a life-or-death decision.

My body is the greatest healing machine, given the proper nutrition. In 1 Corinthians 6:19-20, Paul sums it up concisely, "Do you not know that your body is the temple of the Holy Spirit, who is in you, whom you have received from God? You are not your own: you were bought at a price. Therefore honor God with your body." I did not honor God with my body by consuming so much fat, salt, and sugar, or by gaining 65 lbs. and a host of heart-related ailments. Obesity is not honoring God with your body, yet studies suggest nearly two-thirds of adults are obese.

When I chose to live, I also chose to be as healthy as possible. I still don't always get it right. I'll slip up now and then, but I get right back to it. I am convinced that eating nutritiously has played a significant role in my recovery and extending my life.

Honor God with your body to stay off that heart transplant list. Pray, have some faith, eat healthfully, and decide to live your life *today*. Life is fragile, and time's up.

Afterword

Yesterday, the Sanger Clinic called. They said they were taking me off the transplant list because tests show the condition of my heart has improved. To say I am elated, thankful, and blessed would be an understatement. I continue to be overwhelmed by the grace of God. I have known since June 11, 2009, that God has had me firmly in His grasp. Even when times were tough, the news was not great, and my flesh demanded I let go of God, He never let go of me. He has you firmly in His grasp and whether you like it or not, think it or not, feel it or not, or believe it or not, He will never let go of you either!

In the words of the awesome Apostle Paul, "For I am convinced that neither death nor life, neither angels nor demons, neither the present nor the future, nor any powers, neither height nor depth, nor anything else in all creation, will be able to separate us from the love of God that is in Christ Jesus our Lord." (Romans 8:38-39) And I would also like to add: neither will heart disease, cancer, divorce, depression, unemployment, or high gas prices. God has it all covered.

I look forward to what is ahead, but I am constantly reminded to live each moment as it comes.

God Bless, Art
March 3, 2011

www.ingramcontent.com/pod-product-compliance
Lightning Source LLC
LaVergne TN
LVHW011419080426
835512LV00005B/156